Your Time to Thrive

Your Time to Thrive

Five Keys to Optimizing Health at Any Age

Dr. Adam Dombrowski, ND, LAc and
Dr. Krista Imre, ND

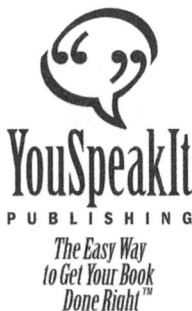

YouSpeakIt

PUBLISHING

*The Easy Way
to Get Your Book
Done Right*™

ISBN: 978-1-957972-10-7

This book is dedicated to those who realize that while a healthy person has a million wishes, a sick person only has one wish.

Contents

Acknowledgments

Thank you to:

All our family and friends who supported our journey to become doctors who practice medicine that *goes against the grain*.

All the mentors, coaches, and teachers who have helped us to become the best practitioners we can be.

The entire staff at Freedom Practice Coaching, who have helped us to create a life-changing practice.

The nonexclusive spirit of the universe, which provides us all the capacity for this precious life.

Introduction

If you live with one or more chronic health concerns, feel stuck in the hamster wheel of conventional medicine, and are not offered anything more than five minutes and a handful of pills per medical visit, then this is the book for you.

This book is about seizing the opportunity to change your health and how to thrive rather than just survive.

This book is also about you; it helps you understand how you arrived where you are now and what led you to your current state of health. This is why we start by painting the big picture, discussing how our country has become a place where many people are unwell.

This book will help you discover the vision for your health and what you want for your life. It helps you identify where you want to go. If you don't know where you're going, you won't know how to get there.

Once you've established your destination, you need an understanding of how to get there and how to change your situation. To accomplish this, you must take control of the biggest factors determining true health, which we call the Pillars of Health. The Pillars are the common threads applied to the healing process for all types of disease.

We define each of these Pillars and explain how they can either create health or, if ignored, create disease. Think of yourself or a friend or loved one who is struggling with their health; the absence of these Pillars will contribute to their suffering consistently and without fail. On the flip side, the proper application of the Pillars will contribute to their healing. This is how we know that our health is always getting better or getting worse. It is never staying the same.

Which is it going to be for you?

You will also find an action step at the end of each chapter. This will allow you to start making tangible changes in your health and life immediately. Each step is a recommendation of how you can put the Pillars of Health into practice. Do not let those opportunities go to waste.

What is knowledge without action? Act on what you learn.

We also discuss the common thread of inflammation throughout these disease patterns and how the Pillars of Health help address dysfunctional inflammation. Patterns of inflammation are common throughout most disease types, including conditions that are the leading cause of disability and mortality. This includes cardiovascular disease, cancer, type 2 diabetes, chronic kidney disease, nonalcoholic fatty liver disease, autoimmune conditions, and neurodegenerative disorders (Hunter 2012; Furman 2019).

On the flip side, this means that balancing inflammation will contribute to healing.

Since we are coauthoring this book, I am going to talk about myself, Dr. Adam, and my colleague, Dr. Krista, who helped me formulate these ideas. We are both naturopathic doctors. I have further training as a licensed acupuncturist, and Dr. Krista as a certified Ayurvedic health specialist. *Ayurveda* is the ancient medicinal philosophy of India. Our functional medical training has helped us to end needless suffering not only in our own lives, but also in the lives of thousands of others.

For Dr. Krista, this is a deeply personal story. When she was a teenager, she was diagnosed with *polycystic ovarian syndrome* (PCOS). This condition got in the way of living her life—causing acne, menstrual issues, unwanted hair growth, and weight gain—leaving her insecure and unwell. To manage her condition, she would have had to take medication for the rest of her life.

After hearing that from her medical doctor, she decided that was unacceptable. She felt as though her body had betrayed her as a young teenager, and now her only option was to medicate for the rest of her life. She was even told she would have to take more medications if she ever wanted to get pregnant. She knew there must be a better way. That led her to discover naturopathic medicine—a better way indeed.

My story is about my father who was diagnosed with a rare autoimmune neurodegenerative disease called *chronic inflammatory demyelinating polyneuropathy* or CIDP. As a result, the muscles in the back of his legs and glutes have withered away such that he cannot use those muscles, so he has trouble walking and was forced to stop playing basketball, a sport that he loved dearly. His conventional doctors could only offer medication and intravenous treatments, which likely slowed the progression of the disease, but these certainly were not helping him to get better.

His conventional doctors were not discussing his lifestyle, sleep, stress levels, what he ate, or other factors that might have been causing his symptoms. Their approach was limited. It was not until my training in functional medicine that I was able to help my father. We changed his lifestyle habits and finally saw positive changes occurring. As a result, he is able to ride his bicycle every day. He has always loved to be super-active, so he is incredibly grateful to have that pleasure and satisfaction again.

This is why we do what we do.

We wrote this book to pass on this hidden knowledge to you and fulfill our vision of reducing unnecessary suffering in the world.

We recommend two things so you can get the most out of this reading.

First, read this book within an ideal mindset and setting. As for *mindset*, you want to be relaxed with the intention that you are doing something good for yourself and for your health. The *setting*, the environment you are in, is the other piece.

When you settle in to read, find a quiet space where you can focus with as little distraction as possible, a space conducive to getting the most you can get out of this book, because this may be the most important book you ever read. That is no exaggeration. These ideas make the difference between health and sickness, between a fulfilling life and a substandard life, and in the most severe cases, literally between life and death.

Second, as you continue reading this book, remember that everything is connected. This viewpoint varies from conventional medicine, in which the body and its care are divided into separate pieces, so you go see one specialist for your liver, another for your joints, and another for your heart and lungs. These doctors are specialists in their field, but that is not how the body works. Everything is connected.

So, while this book is separated into chapters regarding various components of health, they are all connected. We cannot leave any of them out, and you cannot apply them separately. Seeing specialists will not help you nearly as much as integrating everything together into one cohesive, unified whole. Of course, if one of the chapters stands out and you think: *This is the missing piece for me*, or *I haven't heard about this before, and I want to learn more,* then yes, you should dive in and learn more. But remember, without all the other chapters, you will not have the full picture.

Our hope for you is that you gain an understanding of what has been missing in your current approach to health. You'll learn why the Pillars of Health are necessary toward your goal of optimizing your well-being and balancing inflammation. Finally, you'll have an idea of which Pillars you need to address in your own life; and as a result, you'll recognize that all this knowledge will be meaningless if you don't act.

CHAPTER ONE

A Better Approach to Your Health

WHERE DOES YOUR PATH TO HEALTH LEAD?

If you and I were to sit face to face, I would tell you this book is about your life and the quality of every moment you live. Your health is inseparable from your life experience. Maybe you have persistent fatigue preventing you from work or play, and sometimes it's so bad that you can't sleep or relax without feeling exhausted. Perhaps being overweight isn't helping you enjoy various activities with your friends and family.

I don't want to be around people right now.

Perhaps you've been diagnosed with diabetes, thyroid disease, high blood pressure or high cholesterol, or autoimmune or inflammatory disease and don't want to rely on medications.

The doctor said there's nothing else I can do; I must take this medication for life.

You might be going through menopause or andropause—the male counterpart to female menopause—and having a rough time.

Well, I'm getting old. What did I expect?

Maybe you feel trapped in a never-ending cycle of stress and anxiety, or you've always felt deep down there is a better way to live.

Feeling heavy, tired, anxious, and depressed can't be normal, right?

Maybe you are not terribly sick, but you are not where you want to be.

I don't feel as good as I used to feel; I know there is more to life than this.

If any of this is true, then this book is for you. And here is the good news: Your body doesn't hopelessly break down over time. No, your body retains the absolute power to both heal itself and maintain optimal health. The trick is building the right foundation no matter what health concerns you are dealing with, and that is not limited to those concerns listed above.

This reminds me of our practice member, a middle-aged, married woman named Caron. When she started, she said: *I was a mess.* She was addicted to sugar, sleeping poorly, and had difficulty beginning her day. This was compounded with daily digestive problems like acid reflux, gas, and bloating. Over-the-counter antacids and other drugs weren't helping.

Skeptical, she had many questions at first, but she knew her current approach wasn't working and that she needed to do something different. After three months, she recognized the value of a holistic approach. She had no more digestive issues, eliminated her need for blood pressure medication, experienced refreshing sleep, and finally remembered what being energetic felt like. She also lost ten pounds, which wasn't a major goal, but it was a confidence boost. She now looks forward to what each day brings rather than *dragging herself out of bed* each morning.

Being Honest With Yourself

Your health is either getting better or worse, never staying the same, as you navigate life. You can ultimately choose one path or the other, but the first step is recognizing which path you are currently on.

1. **Get Clear**.

   Ask yourself: *Am I truly maintaining a healthy lifestyle?*

   Be brutally honest with yourself. There is nothing to gain from avoiding the truth.

   It is also crucial to look at yourself in the mirror and have enough integrity to be honest about your life, the one precious life that you have the opportunity to live.

Be honest with yourself about what condition you are in as you observe yourself:

How do you feel in your current life?

Perform an audit of your daily emotional patterns. Compare whether you generally have more good days or more bad days, and on those bad days, what are your points of greatest suffering?

Consider your mind, body, and spirit.

What do you wish was better or different?

Take time to spell that out for yourself—it is absolutely pivotal. It is akin to making the correct diagnosis. Any treatment options are ultimately irrelevant if we don't have the correct diagnosis.

Once you have clarity, move to the second step.

2. **Make a Choice**.

Ask: *Is my health important enough to make a better decision for myself, to find a better way and step on the path I desire?*

Don't overanalyze this—a simple yes or no will suffice. Again, brutal honesty is crucial here.

I may not know what it is like to have diabetes, be overweight, have chronic fatigue, or take multiple medications, but I do know what it is like to struggle. Suffering comes in many forms. For me, it was severe social anxiety and emotional insecurity.

I specifically remember one time, as a teenager, eating at a pizza shop with my family. After finishing my first slice, I said, "I want a second slice."

My dad threw his arm around me and said, "Great, go up there and order yourself a slice."

I completely froze. A tidal wave of fear and anxiety swelled up inside of me. At that time in my life, I could not speak to anyone I was not familiar with due to this ever-present dread. I couldn't even order a slice of pizza! I absolutely hated being paralyzed by anxiety, not knowing what was causing it and not knowing what to do about it.

But if I had any hope to change, I first had to admit to myself that I was struggling. That was the first step in starting my transformation to achieve a better life, to improve my mental and emotional well-being, and eventually discover more freedom in social situations. If I hadn't had the courage to admit that to myself, I would never have changed, and I cannot imagine what life would be like now.

I know what it is like to struggle; emotional symptoms are a sign of *dis-ease* just like any other organic disease, e.g., diabetes, thyroid disorder, chronic fatigue, and so on. That is why I am so passionate about creating better health and why I want the same for you. I want you to experience the same freedom of life I and so many of our practice members experience. I want you to break out of the cage, knowing there is a better life within reach.

Health Affects Your Life, Your Family, Your Work

Now that you are being honest with yourself, it is important to discern how the state of your health is affecting your life. Think about all areas of life here—maybe you do not have the energy to get out of bed, to go up and down the stairs, or fold your laundry. You are lethargic or moody and don't want to be around people. This can cause small day-to-day activities to feel burdensome and keep you from traveling or going on a hike with family or friends.

Maybe you feel too depressed to go on vacation, too tired to have fun. But think about how it affects your loved ones, your family and friends who do not get to spend time with you because you don't feel well. You can't maximize your time with your kids or spouse because you are not feeling well.

Achieving your optimal health is not for you alone; it is also for your friends, family, children, and loved ones. You become a role model for your children, to raise them well and experience those landmark moments in their life. You can enjoy life with your spouse and maybe travel together with your best friends because you have energy. You can roll around on the floor freely with your grandkids or your pets and feel confident enough to go to the beach and feel good in your bathing suit.

These four questions can help you find your way:

- What about your life currently do you not like?

- How might your health concerns be holding you back?

- Why do you not like your current situation and want to change it?

- What more do you want in life and why?

Consider not only what you want to *have* and what you want to *do*, but also how you want to *feel*. This will clarify what you want to change and why.

Use the space below to record your replies:

Your answers to the above questions together define your *why*, your motivation to reach the carrot at the end of the stick. Knowing your *why* is the force to propel you through difficult and challenging moments as they arise while you pursue a different path to a better life. This can be difficult for some people to answer, but I hope you now know yours. If not, go back, grab a pen, and do this exercise before reading onward.

Nancy was a forty-year-old, full-time mother whose health concerns were disrupting her everyday life. She began her days feeling sluggish and couldn't take care of her kids as abundantly as she wanted to. Preparing her kids for school and handling simple personal affairs was incredibly effortful. Her symptoms also prevented her from working and earning income. Brain fog didn't make the days any easier. She was also fearful of developing cancer, as it ran in her family, so she wanted to do everything she could to prevent it.

She saw herself as generally healthy and thought her concerns might be due to motherhood stress or possibly her *age*. In her own efforts to solve her health issues, she did research, but was consistently overwhelmed with conflicting information, leaving her with more questions than answers.

After seeking professional guidance and following a customized approach addressing the root cause of her concerns, she is tremendously relieved to have her life back, and she can finally be the type of mother she wants to be.

Nancy reports: *Now I get out of bed with a bounce, and I feel so energized to get my day started, and I can keep going all day without getting exhausted. I'm in a great mood and happy, feeling in control of my life and health. I am a fun mom rather than a* cranky mom. *Overall, my program was life-changing for both myself and my whole family. Feeling healthy . . . and an abundance of energy is priceless!*

It Doesn't Have to Be That Way

Your current path is leading you somewhere you do not want to be. You may have been told by your doctor: *Well, you are getting older, what do you expect?* or *There is nothing else you can do, just take the medication, and come back if anything gets worse.*

That is the conventional approach, and it probably leaves you discouraged. You are not alone. Many experience this sense of hopelessness when seeking help. The current healthcare system is more so a system of disease management, that is, *managing the disease* to help you survive rather than thrive.

It is possible to thrive because we have seen this time and time again with our practice members, with people who are willing to find the proper guidance and make necessary changes. It is never too late to make a change for your health, a change for the better. If you recognize your current approach is not working, are willing to step outside of that approach, and can commit to the vision of what you truly want, then there is hope.

You cannot afford to wait until it is too late. Allowing your health to run unchecked raises your odds of developing a worst-case diagnosis and spending your time, money, and energy being in and out of hospitals. Sometimes we consult with a person who chooses not to take action on their health, and six months down the road, their health has only gotten worse.

Good health will not simply fall into your lap, but the good news is that good health can be created.

In February of 2018, my Aunt Joanie was diagnosed with that scary word nobody wants to hear: *cancer*. For her it was liver cancer that spread to her lungs and bones, and she was given about a year to live. My Aunt Joanie was overweight, extremely fatigued, and deeply depressed. She suffered from widespread joint pain. This kept her chained to her couch almost all day. She never left her house, except for dragging herself to the hospital every week or two for rounds of cancer treatment, occasional surgery, and regular blood draws and to see her team of specialists.

Compare this to my Aunt Joanie twenty years prior—vibrant, full of energy, a social butterfly who absolutely loved to dance. It was around this time that her health began showing early signs of illness, e.g., low mood, low energy, arthritic pain, and so on. Her life was now essentially reduced to watching television and speaking to us by phone every other day. The multiple medications she took for depression and pain barely took the edge off. She experienced much more suffering than she did comfort.

As a result of all this, my family and I could no longer enjoy her company because she was no longer able to come over for holidays. It saddens us because we have great memories with her, but that is all we will likely ever have. We all wish there were something different my aunt could have done that would have led to different results.

I firmly believe there was. Had she been open to a new approach and been willing to make any changes with her life, starting with those early symptoms and signs of ill health, I know it would have dramatically impacted her health and changed the trajectory of her life. I can tell you she never would have picked up and read a book like this.

Do not wait until it is too late. Pat yourself on the back, keep reading, and remember to act before the opportunity to change slips away.

Skip to the last page of this book if you'd like to act right now or at any point you feel inspired throughout this reading.

Start now. Your life and loved ones depend on it.

LIMITS OF THE CONVENTIONAL APPROACH

Here are some statistics that illustrate the current efficacy of the United States healthcare system:

- In 2019, the annual cost of healthcare in the United States was $3.8 trillion (American Medical Association). Ninety percent of that amount was spent on the management of chronic health conditions (Buttorff, Ruder, and Bauman 2017; Martin et al. 2020).

- Chronic diseases are defined as conditions present for more than one year that also limit activities of daily living or require ongoing medical care. These are common diseases, including heart disease, diabetes, cancer, obesity, stroke, Alzheimer's, chronic kidney disease, and arthritis.

- Six out of ten adults in the United States have one chronic disease and four out of ten have two or more (Centers for Disease Control and Prevention A).

- The five most common chronic diseases—heart disease, cancer, stroke, chronic obstructive pulmonary disease, and diabetes—together account for more than 70 percent of all deaths, or 1.7 million Americans every year (Tinker 2017).

- People who are reported to be in the poorest category of health, most of whom are affected by these top chronic diseases, have average healthcare expenditures of $26,450 per person per year (Nunn 2020).

- In comparison to eleven high-income countries, the U.S. ranks last in overall healthcare performance, despite spending far more on health care. It specifically ranks last on both access to care and health care outcomes (Schneider et al. 2021).

The basic responsibility of the healthcare system is to meet the needs of current illnesses and patients. Clearly, the system is lacking something significant. For a healthcare system that spends more per person than any other country, the United States should be ranked much higher.

One of the biggest problems that leads to these poor outcomes is that patients are not taught how to achieve control and responsibility of their own health. Instead, they fully discharge that responsibility to the doctor, the medication, the surgery, and so on, believing that the only way to get better is to rely on external support or luck.

You do have control over your health and life. Age and genetics do not dictate everything; they are only part of the story. A rising field called *Epigenetics* describes how much lifestyle controls genetic expression, so much so that you can turn the tide of your own health. That's right—every one of your choices and behaviors actually changes the way your DNA expresses itself.

Your health cannot afford to wait for prescriptions and procedures to save you. Take ownership of your life and place yourself on the path to empowerment. At the time of this writing, the COVID-19 pandemic has been present for two full years with no end in sight. This global event is characterized by widespread fear of the virus. Much of this fear stems from the belief that people do not have control over their health. Now, we know that outcomes to COVID-19 are typically worse in people with multiple chronic health problems, many of them are reversible. This does not only apply to COVID-19, but also other threats to our health, such as bacterial infections or the seasonal flu.

While there will always be situations out of your control, you can control your health. This will not only prevent deterioration of your health, but also increase your vitality and strengthen your resilience to a potential infection. That is what the rest of this book is about.

Pills

Many people believe their primary care practitioner, the person wearing the white coat, has all the answers they need. They think the solution to their struggle comes in a prescription bottle. They take the pill(s) prescribed by their doctor and expect all will be well. However, this approach is very limited for two reasons. First, everyone with the same symptoms gets the same type of medication, a *cookie-cutter* approach. Second, the medication usually fails to address the true cause of the symptom.

To illustrate this idea of symptom versus cause, let's look at high blood pressure as an example. If you see you have high numbers when checking your blood pressure and take blood pressure medication, will that lower your blood pressure? Yes, it will. But what happens if you were to stop taking the blood pressure medication? Your blood pressure would climb again. There is clearly an underlying cause that has not been addressed, something missing as part of the equation. You must discover the cause if you don't want to rely on medication anymore.

Another analogy is the indicator light on your car. If the light on the dashboard turns on, this specifies there is an issue somewhere within the vehicle. To fix the problem, would you snip the wire to the light on your dashboard to turn it off and call the problem fixed? Of course not! There is clearly an underlying problem remaining deeper in the automobile system that needs to be addressed. This is where the help of a trained professional becomes valuable, someone who knows what to look for. Snipping the wire to turn off the dashboard light is ignoring the problem, not solving it. This may create a sense of temporary relief, but in the long term, it will be detrimental.

Health does not come in a prescription bottle. We all wish that could be true, but it's not the reality. Medication and surgery, while they are important to prevent dangerous health issues such as heart attack or stroke, lead to short-term results rather than long-term resolutions. Since you are reading this book, I assume this is the kind of approach you don't want. You are likely here because you want long-term resolution, and you're in the right place.

Procedures

While they have their place in medicine, pills and procedures are both things we hope you do not need. Like medication, medical procedures also typically serve to manage the symptom and not treat the cause. Unfortunately, these are the only tools many doctors have in their toolbox, so that is all they know how to use. As they say: *When you have a hammer, everything you see is a nail.*

So it is with a surgical physician; when they discover a problem, say a tumor growth or an orthopedic issue, they are inclined to suggest a procedure, like total knee replacement surgery or incision to remove a tumor growth from the body, without considering the deeper cause of these issues.

Like the car analogy above, you do not want to resort to removing parts of your engine because something is wrong with the way the car drives. The parts are there for a reason. There might be an issue elsewhere in the body that could explain the problem.

Choosing a different path and finding a mentor with a more holistic perspective will benefit you. Before resorting to drastic measures, consider a comprehensive evaluation by a more holistic practitioner before any drastic moves are made. In medicine, for example, many patients have inflammatory conditions affecting their intestine or gall bladder, and often, physicians suggest the removal of the problematic organ. Removal is usually not your only option.

If you identify the cause, then you can find a way to address it, and the inflammatory issue may resolve as a result. Besides, every organ has a purpose and removing one will impair your body's natural function in a way associated to that organ's purpose.

Pills and procedures are a *backup* plan for use in urgent circumstances. If you have emergent high blood pressure and need to lower it quickly, that is what medications and procedures are for. While this short-sighted perspective serves a purpose and is necessary for high-risk and emergent situations, it is not reliable and effective for long-term treatment.

Mary, another full-time mom, was always putting others before herself, and her health suffered as a result. She saw no way out of her intolerable situation. She felt stuck in the conventional medical system. Every time she went to the doctor, she was given a new medication. She was eventually taking eight medications, including a monthly injection mostly to manage her chronic hives. She also had fatigue, headaches, menstrual pain that radiated down her legs, weight gain, and an autoimmune disorder called *Hashimoto's*. There had to be a way to heal without hopelessly relying on more medications. This was unacceptable to both her and her husband. They knew there had to be a way to resolve this without hopelessly relying on more medications.

That is why she committed to a different approach, an individualized, holistic approach that focused on the root causes of her condition. As a result, six months later, she was off most medications and had decreased the last one—no more miserable hives, headaches, and menstrual pains. She had energy to guide her through the day, for herself and her kids. She even lost fifty pounds. She planted the right foundations, and these foundations helped her body to finally heal itself.

Insurance

Think about the people around you.

You will see that many people are not getting better. Instead, they are becoming increasingly sick. Unfortunately, patients and wellness are not at the center focus of the healthcare-insurance system. Regrettably, this is partly because most healthcare decisions are made based on money. There is too much financial and political influence involved, so it is sad but true that healthcare decisions often come down to the *almighty dollar*. Pharmaceutical companies spend billions of dollars on advertising, and health insurance companies try to maximize profit.

Should insurance have paid for a program like what Mary went through? Of course, they should—but do they? No.

Health insurance should also pay for natural treatments that have substantial clinical support for their efficacy and reliability, but it does not. Your insurance company likely pays for only pills and procedures; they pay for the things we hope you do not need.

Health insurance should really be called *sick insurance* because it is not there to improve your health. The purpose of insurance is to help manage problems that arise, to help with damage control. It does not help you to optimize your situation. Like pills and procedures, most health insurance programs do not help you get better. They are designed only to keep you from becoming worse. You don't want to rely on insurance for your health strategy because by the time you need to draw on it, you are needing to mediate downside rather than finding opportunities to gain upside.

Your car insurance and home insurance work the same way: You cannot rely on insurance to dig you out of the hole you are in. The traditional health insurance model has its place, again for urgent situations, but in the long term, it keeps you stuck in the hamster wheel of conventional medicine. If you are going to escape the hamster wheel and get to the promised land, then you must be willing to step outside the broken system.

THERE IS HOPE

You may feel frustrated or discouraged about your health. You are not alone. Most people with seemingly endless struggles are also fed up. Even healthcare practitioners are frustrated. They see the lack of results using the conventional approach to medicine. They are not able to help their patients as they expect, and they do not know how to achieve better results or are not able to go outside of what insurance dictates and covers.

Because we have seen so many people suffering with chronic health issues, we also know that many of these people have turned their health around. It is possible for you to find a better way and to take control. To pursue that hope, you must be willing to break through the barrier of fear and discomfort that might result from a different and unfamiliar approach.

Along with the support of what you will learn in this book, always remember your *why*, which you defined earlier. That fire burning will light your way through to the other side of that barrier.

Treating the Cause, Not Just the Symptoms

By now you know that if we are going to lead you to your desired destination, then you must be willing to put in the work. However, we first need to uncover the cause of your symptoms. Most physicians in conventional settings are allotted very little time with each patient, and they order only basic tests because this is all that insurance will cover.

This is simply not enough.

Instead of a cookie-cutter approach, you need a customized one. You deserve to be evaluated as a unique individual with unique physiology, all within your unique life. Find a practitioner who is going to prioritize spending enough time with you to learn the unique details of your case. This also means the need for a different approach to testing.

Most doctors perform relatively shallow testing—again, to help ensure there is nothing urgently wrong with your health, that there is no impending doom they need to manage. These tests are the bare minimum, very surface level. Instead, we need to do much more comprehensive testing that is going to help shed light on the cause of your condition.

A practitioner who is trained in a functional approach to health and wellness will have a more holistic view of the body. This typically means they do two things conventional physicians do not: First, they order more in-depth testing; and secondly, they interpret the results properly.

One example of the importance of ordering comprehensive testing is the thyroid. If you have a thyroid condition, then your doctor will look at TSH, which stands for *thyroid stimulating hormone*. This single marker is a basic test that is important, but it provides only a limited picture. There are many more tests for thyroid markers needed, because looking at TSH alone may tell you your thyroid is normal when other markers might indicate dysfunction.

Regarding the way those results are interpreted, you must first understand how the reference ranges are determined. Laboratory reference ranges involve minimum and maximum values. If your result lies within that range, then your result is said to be *normal*. If it falls outside of that range, then the result is considered *abnormal*. But how are these ranges determined in the first place? Well, they are created by studying the average person who gets testing done. This generally means sick people, as healthy people aren't often having tests run.

Let me ask you: Is the average population a healthy population? No, we have already discussed that. Unfortunately, it is more common to be unwell than it is to be well. It is more common to be unhealthy and taking multiple medications than it is to be thriving and empowered with your health without a reliance on medication.

Let's not confuse *average* with *normal*. It may be average to be sick and unwell, but that does not mean it is normal. Functional doctors understand this; that is why they use "functional reference ranges" instead. These ranges are based on a healthy population—a group of people who are thriving and feeling well. This way you can compare yourself to healthy people, not to average people.

Take the thyroid/TSH example; a TSH result may seem normal to a conventional doctor, but not normal to a functional practitioner. A functional practitioner may see a suboptimal result, indicating an opportunity to optimize thyroid function that may have been contributing to symptoms, though undetected by conventional means. This applies to many other chronic health conditions as well.

Finding a Trustworthy and Accurate Source of Information

There is an abundance of information about health in the world, especially on the internet and from conversations with the people in your life. Health misinformation spreads like wildfire. It is everywhere, so it becomes difficult to separate truth from fiction.

How do we find truth?

How do we find the correct information that will help turn your health around, so you do not waste time and money on this cleanse or that detox or this diet or that supplement?

Supplements can be particularly misleading considering the supplement industry is currently unregulated. As a result, there are a lot of fad supplements. Any company can put nearly anything into a supplement and sell it. They can make certain claims that may not necessarily be true. You must know where to turn to find accurate information.

When searching for a healthcare practitioner, find someone you trust who can sift through everything to find what is most relevant to you.

The Pillars of Health

Ninety-four percent of all failure comes from not having a system (Andrew 2018). In addition to finding a holistic practitioner, you'll also need a proven system to ensure the best results, which will last the rest of your life. Our approach involves a system for evaluating and addressing the root cause of disease. We call that system *The Pillars of Health*. There are five pillars:

- Detoxification
- Nutrition
- Hormones
- Energy regulation
- Mentorship

Everything about your health depends on a solid foundation. If any of those Pillars are missing, your health will become compromised and you will likely struggle to feel well. On the flipside, when these five Pillars are in place, then true health will naturally arise. Add these five Pillars together and you have the picture of true health. This is the simple truth.

The Five Pillars of Health are how we are going to break out of the broken system and address the root cause so you can have ever-lasting wellness. Next, we dive into the meaning of each Pillar, beginning with detoxification, and explain how they can create either disease or health.

Action Item

Write down your answers to the following questions:

- What about your life now do you not like?

- How might your health concerns be holding you back?

- Why do you want to change?

- What more do you want in life? Consider not only what you want to have and what you want to do, but also how you want to feel.

Get clear on your *why*. This will be related to the very last question mentioned above.

CHAPTER TWO

The Importance of Detoxification

TOXINS, STRESS, AND INFLAMMATION

You live in a toxic world.

The consumer culture, which drives the current economy, produces goods on an incredibly immense scale. This production creates byproducts, not all of which are safe. In fact, many are known to be harmful to you. Your health is not at the focus of the world's economic activity—the profit motive is—and this motive comes at your expense. Again, it all comes back to money.

A toxin is any substance that disrupts the normal function of your body, typically causing harm and triggering inflammation.

These toxins essentially exert stress in your body and, like any stress, too much for too long can create lasting issues for your health.

A Toxic World – Three Types of Stress

Let's first put stress in context:

Your body has a baseline of normal function. That balance—the balance of health—can be thrown off by stress of various kinds. These physiological imbalances lead to symptoms, diseases, and conditions. You need to help your body maintain or restore its state of balance by managing sources of stress and the body's response to it.

There are three ways in which your body can experience stress.

1. **Chemical Stress**

   Present in your everyday life, chemical stress is what you normally think of when you think of toxins. Some examples are:

   • Pesticides in food

   • Heavy metals and pollution in the environment

   • Bisphenol A (BPA) in plastic food containers, water bottles, electronics

- Phthalates in personal hygiene products, such as feminine care products

These chemicals throw a wrench into the gears of your health, hampering your body's ability to function.

Some chemicals are *endocrine disruptors*, meaning they block your hormone activity, which puts you at risk for development of a variety of diseases, including:

- Certain cancers
- Autoimmune disease
- Alzheimer's
- Parkinson's
- Hormonal imbalances
- Asthma
- ADHD and other learning differences in children

These chemical toxins can also affect our metabolism, creating conditions like diabetes and obesity (Schug et al. 2011).

2. **Physical Stress**

This includes physical exertion of or impact to your body. Sometimes that means a car accident or another injurious impact to the body. It also refers to physical activity—manual labor, housework, or exercise. Not all physical stress is bad, right? Exercise and manual work are good for the body. However, doing too much of it or performing it with improper technique can create stress on the body and damage tissues. Such excessive or improper use can also create muscular weakness or structural misalignments that may lead to chronic pain in muscles, tendons, and joints.

3. **Emotional Stress**

This is what most people think of when they hear the word *stress*. Of course, we all know the feeling of inner tension and angst that stress can cause. When we experience emotional stress from our jobs, friends, or family, there are two parts of your nervous system involved:

- Sympathetic Nervous System

The sympathetic nervous system is responsible for the fight or flight response. This causes your heart to beat faster. You become anxious, alert, warm, and sweaty and energy flows to your muscles. The purpose of these physiological reactions is to deal with a stressful event. Evolutionarily, mammals have had occasional life-threatening encounters, like seeing a tiger appear, and the body would need to prepare to either fight or run. These physiological responses are the essential feeling of stress we all experience.

- Parasympathetic Nervous System

The other aspect of your nervous system is the parasympathetic nervous system, which does the opposite. Instead of fight or flight, it helps you rest and digest. When you relax, blood flows to your digestive system instead of your muscles, so you can absorb energy from your food. Your heartbeat also slows, your body temperature decreases to a comfortable degree, and brain chemicals that help you feel calm, cool, and collected are released. However, during times of emotional stress, this parasympathetic system turns down, while the sympathetic system turns up. This is all to say that emotional stress is very tangible; it creates substantial physiological change in your nervous system.

Now remember, as we said, not all stress is bad. Stress is how your body adapts to the environment and becomes stronger. Exercise is physical stress, which is needed to help your body become strong and to maintain that strength. Similarly, some chemical and emotional stress keeps our immune and nervous systems healthy. The problem is most people have excessive exposure to each of these three types of stress, and without a way to mitigate it, their health suffers.

Inflammation

Like stress, inflammation is generally beneficial, unless it becomes excessive. Inflammation is the body's natural mechanism for healing and protecting itself against injuries, infections, and other assaults on your health. Inflammation is essentially a reaction by your immune system to provide healing resources for your body to use.

Imagine if you scraped your leg. The first information your brain receives is that it hurts, which serves a purpose. Pain is your body drawing your attention to that area to ensure you don't damage it further.

Next the affected region becomes red and warm and swollen, which is a sign of your body bringing blood flow to the area. With blood flow come healing resources. The blood carries the immune cells, red blood cells, clotting factors, and nutrients required for healing the wound on your leg. Over the next day or two, you'll see a scab form over the area, as new skin slowly forms underneath. A few days later, the wound is healed. Amazingly, your body does this naturally and automatically—you do not have to think about it.

What else can trigger inflammation? Once inside your body, viruses, bacteria, mold, parasites, or even nonorganic materials can cause an inflammatory response when your body detects that they shouldn't be there. Emotional stress and hormone imbalances also cause a cascade of swelling in your body.

There are two other ways to understand inflammation: *external and internal.* The scrape on your leg is external, visible on the surface of your body, and you can see it. But inflammation can also be internal, where you cannot see it so well. This can make it more difficult to discover without some investigation.

The second dynamic to understand is *acute and chronic*. The inflammatory process can either be short lived, which we call *acute*, or it can be long lasting, which we call *chronic*. The scrape on your leg is an acute inflammatory response since it happens over the course of hours to days and then resolves. A chronic inflammatory response is launched when some virus or bacteria causes short-term issues with acute inflammation, such as bronchitis, pneumonia, or a cold. But many microbes can also linger in the body even after your initial symptoms disappear, leading to long-term issues like Lyme disease or Epstein-Barr virus.

Whether your inflammation is acute or chronic, it is meant to resolve naturally, on its own. But as is the case with many health concerns and conditions, inflammation can last for months or years without resolving. This happens because the cause of inflammation has not been dealt with. In this case, your immune system and stress response have been activated, and your body is stuck in a perpetual cycle. To finally resolve the inflammation, we need to address the underlying trigger.

Connecting Your Symptoms and Conditions

Injury, toxins, microbes, and various forms of stress are common causes of inflammation. When the inflammation is produced, it causes symptoms and diseases. In fact, virtually every chronic condition can be tied to a dynamic of uncontrolled inflammation.

Among the most common are:

- Cancer
- Heart disease
- Diabetes
- Asthma
- Alzheimer's disease
- Arthritis

There are many more, and almost any chronic disease likely counts here. As a result of their chronic issue, most people end up as we discussed in Chapter One—relying on medication to manage their condition, but never arriving at the root cause of their disease pattern.

The truth is that these various forms of stress, toxic exposures, and resulting inflammation often cause chronic disease patterns. Instead of relying solely on medication to manage the symptoms, we want to get to the root cause of these diseases and address them completely. We want to help your body release toxins so your body can naturally heal itself, and that will happen only if all obstacles are cleared.

So how does your body get rid of toxins and inflammation naturally?

It is equipped with a natural mechanism called *detoxification*.

DETOXIFICATION

Detoxification is a natural process your body carries out on its own. Because we live in a toxic world, the body is vulnerable to toxic exposure and other negative influences. At the same time, your body is dynamic, resilient, and strong and has a way to protect you against these toxins.

Detoxification is not something you do once. Many people undertake a *detox* for a week and then are done with it. They do it once a year, or maybe once in a lifetime, and that's all. That is not the right idea.

Understand that your body is undergoing a natural detoxification process every minute of every day, as reliably as your lungs breathe and your heart beats. Your detox organs—primarily the gut, liver, kidneys, and skin—are continually eliminating toxins to maintain optimal health. Problems arise when those organs are not taken care of, and the resulting dysfunction causes toxins to get backed up in the system.

The Need to Detox

If we do not get rid of toxins regularly, the resulting organ dysfunction can lead to inflammation and various symptoms.

Fortunately, this mechanism for dysfunction can actually become the same mechanism for healing. Because your body is detoxing every minute of every day, supporting your body's ability to detox will rid you of excess toxic load and inflammation. To be clear, we do not want to get rid of inflammation completely; we only want to tone it down when there is too much. Once you have rebalanced your inflammatory process, then your body is able to function normally once again. To accomplish this, your body primarily depends on four organs to detox:

- Liver

  The liver is a large triangular shaped organ protected by your rib cage and is the main hub for filtering your blood. Any toxins entering your body through food, water, and pharmaceutical medications are mostly filtered through your liver.

- Gut

  Then there is the gut; how does the gut get rid of toxins? Through the stool. So having regular and complete bowel movements ensures that your body is ridding itself of toxins.

- Skin

  Next is our skin, where we sweat out toxins. That is why regular exercise and sauna use both support detox.

- Kidneys

Finally, the kidneys flush toxins through the urine. That is why you need to stay hydrated, so your kidneys can use that water to filter out into the urine everything your body does not need.

To keep the toxin load low and allow your immune system a chance to finally tone down the inflammation, these four organs must function effectively. Obviously, we want to keep the toxin load in our body to be low as opposed to high. The body can handle a reasonable amount, but at some point, we hit a threshold. Think of the body as a bucket you fill with water. As you continue filling the bucket, at some point, it overflows.

That is an illustration of a body overburdened by excess toxic load. To keep the metaphor going, we want to keep a small opening at the bottom of the bucket to keep water moving through at a steady pace, and to avoid the bucket from overfilling.

It is not reasonable to expect your bucket to be completely empty, since toxins are omnipresent and will inevitably make their way in, no matter what. But neither do we want our bucket to be so full your body is overwhelmed and unable to handle additional stress. You always want extra space available, so your body has capacity to handle the next unpredictable stress that comes your way.

What Detoxification Is Not

Most people are misinformed about detox. This usually involves following a regimen that uses either suppositories or laxatives, putting you on the toilet for hours each day. This is misguided and unnecessary. Detoxification is not supposed to be unpleasant. Forget about everything that you've previously thought or believed about detox and keep an open mind.

Supporting detox is different from doing a cleanse. A lot of people think these terms are interchangeable, but let's explore how they are different.

While both focus on eating healthy foods, a cleanse is typically focused only on digestive health. Detox support focuses more on the whole person. Detoxification is a systemic approach to toxin removal from the body. The focus is more on how all your organs function together, rather than the digestive system and the intestines. Because of this, it should not leave you feeling crappy like a lot of people expect. They think of someone feeling tired with a headache and flu-like symptoms.

That can happen in certain cases, and if it does, it should not be debilitating. But usually, people still go about their day feeling fine. When approached properly, detox is supposed to leave you feeling refreshed, restored, and re-energized.

What Detoxification Is

Detox is not an event. It is not something you do once a year or season. Rather, your body is always detoxing, so you need to make it a part of your daily lifestyle as a gentle, yet powerful, process.

To accomplish this, you first need to reduce toxic exposure, wherever that may be. Often this relates to those chemical toxins I mentioned earlier, a primary culprit being food, which carries pesticides and artificial or genetically modified ingredients. These turn our food into low-grade poison, placing a burden on the detox capacity of your body and filling your bucket that much more.

Food is one example, but think about the plastic and personal hygiene products mentioned earlier. Once identified, remove them from your life. Toxic exposure also means emotional stress, which increases stress hormones in the body caused by difficult circumstances like an overwhelming job or family situation. I am not telling you to quit your job or leave your family, but consider what you might have control over to change for the better.

Removing toxins from your environment could include:

- Requesting to work more from home

- Swapping home cleaning and personal hygiene products for ones that contain fewer toxic ingredients

- Seeing a relationship counselor

- Discovering games with your children that allow quiet time for Mom and Dad

- Starting a daily meditation practice

It can take some creativity and brainstorming to find solutions that really work for the long term.

Second, we need to help restore function to your detox organs: the gut, liver, skin, and kidneys. When these organs function at their best, they will continue eliminating the ongoing toxic exposure remaining.

We support our detox organs in the following ways:

- Eating real food
- Taking supplements
- Staying well-hydrated
- Exercising regularly
- Sleeping well

This allows inflammation in the body to reduce and rebalance. The reduction of overall inflammation helps your body switch back into parasympathetic mode so healing can resume.

Do you remember the two parts of the nervous system, the sympathetic nervous system and the parasympathetic nervous system? We generally want more parasympathetic activity to stimulate healing. Detoxification helps your body to shift into parasympathetic mode by ridding these toxins rather than being in the fight or flight sympathetic state, where our body is not able to efficiently eliminate toxins and promote healing.

OUR APPROACH TO DETOXIFICATION

You know the difference between a cleanse and a detox. Our approach to detox takes a holistic medical perspective, looking at the entire body, mind, and spirit together. It is not a commercial approach or based on a Dr. Google perspective. It is a professionally guided medical detox. If we want to create maximum results, then we need to work with trained professionals and customize the approach to your unique physiological needs and uniqueness.

Specific Detox Therapies

You may be familiar with some detox therapies, but it is important to understand how they help your body detox.

We talked about the first step of eliminating triggers. This is fundamental because you can see the insanity in forever trying to rid your body of toxins when you have not attempted to fix the source of toxic exposure. This includes eliminating food triggers that may be causing food sensitivities.

A *food sensitivity* is when a specific food creates negative reactions in your body, leading to dysfunction in detox and healing. It is important to figure out what those unique food sensitivities are for you specifically because they are different for everybody. The best diet for you will be different from the best diet for your friend, cousin, or co-worker. Those foods must be identified and removed from the diet.

Food sensitivities are different from food allergies. A *food allergy* is like an anaphylactic reaction, meaning it happens within minutes to hours after you eat the food, so you know which food was the offender. Food sensitivity is different; this type of reaction to a particular food happens over hours to days, so it might not be obvious to you. Still, we must get to the bottom of it.

We also use supplements in an individualized fashion. They may be used to support liver or gall bladder function, heal gut lining, or increase circulation, depending on your needs. Usually, we do a *spring cleaning* initially to help your body clear out the high load of toxins, which, in some cases, has built up over forty to fifty years in people who have not supported detoxification before. We may use more supplements at the start, and then once your body can handle regular detox on its own, a more simple approach can be used.

Another detox therapy is called *hydrotherapy*. It applies heat and cold to the body in different ways. Hydrotherapy is used to:

- Stimulate sweating
- Balance hormones
- Improve both immune and cardiovascular function

- Increase mental clarity
- Increase circulation of lymph, bile, and blood—fluids that carry toxins out of the body

All these benefits also result from fitness, which is why we additionally use various fitness methods to support detox. Hydrotherapy and fitness both help balance your emotions, release stress, and pump your body full of feel-good hormones like endorphins.

These are a few of the methods we use. This is not an all-inclusive list. There are more.

A Personalized Approach

Like any other treatment, there is not a one-size-fits-all, cookie-cutter approach to detox that will work for everybody. Specific therapies vary from person to person, but the principles remain the same. We individualize the process to your unique medical needs, focusing on both safety and effectiveness.

Throughout a detox support process, the reactions you may end up with will be either negative or positive. You will benefit from support; therefore, you need to work with a trained professional. An experienced practitioner will not only guide you through choosing what detox strategies are right for you, but also guide you through the detox experience itself and make appropriate changes along the way. This allows your detox to remain as safe and effective as possible. Otherwise, you cannot expect to get the results you are looking for.

Positive and Negative Experiences

Throughout a detox, people can experience *good* and *bad* reactions.

Unpleasant symptoms may develop, so we must remember that many people have gone for years without detoxing, maybe even their whole life. As a result, and continuing with our bucket metaphor, your bucket could be full—or even over the rim.

As you help your body rid itself of toxins, you may have a poor reaction. This is to be expected considering how many toxins have built up inside your body. When they are finally released and handled, it is not surprising that it doesn't feel good. But you should not have many detox symptoms if you have prepared correctly.

So the question you should ask yourself is: *How do I prepare?*

You prepare by eliminating processed food, sugar, and your unique food sensitivities from your diet. You take measures to heal your gut and get your lymph, bile, and blood circulation moving. However, if you have multiple chronic diseases over a very long time—say ten, twenty, thirty years, or longer—and take a lot of medications, which again add to the toxic burden on the body, this also makes unpleasant reactions less surprising. If this is the case for you, it may mean you'll need a longer preparation period.

Some common reactions to detox:

- Low energy
- Headaches
- Constipation
- Diarrhea
- Bloating
- Brain fog

If these negative reactions do occur, they can be a good sign that toxins are being dumped from the body. We call a reaction like this a *healing reaction*. The reaction is temporary, but it indicates an effort to heal.

Last are the positive reactions to detox. Many people experience increased energy and weight changes. Fat tissue stores toxins and is inflammatory, so when your body is eliminating these toxins, it discharges fat, and inflammation decreases as a result. You'll notice that you start to shed weight, regain your energy, and rebalance your blood. Your mood and energy are better, your skin brightens, and your cravings are either diminished or gone. Many of our practice members generally feel the best during the detox phase.

Action Item

Drink enough water. Your body is majorly dependent on water for getting rid of waste via the numerous detox organs we discussed.

- Hydrate consistently every single day!

- Drink half of your bodyweight in ounces every day (e.g., if you weigh 150 pounds, drink 75 ounces of water each day).

- Strive to be consistent. Urine that appears clear to light yellow signifies you've been drinking enough. Darker urine suggests you should increase your water intake.

Bonus hacks:

- Keep a 1-liter water bottle with you most of the day and aim to drink at least two full bottles daily.

- Adding a solute to the water can help you enjoy drinking and stimulate your desire to do it more often. Add a splash of 100 percent juice, trace mineral drops, or electrolyte powder to enhance the taste.

CHAPTER THREE

The Importance of Nutrition

WHAT IS NUTRITION AND WHY DO WE NEED IT?

Nutrition is an indispensable foundation for your health. It is one of the most beneficial steps you can take to impact your well-being, and if you want to navigate back to peak wellness, you absolutely need to consider what you are eating.

Definition - What Is Nutrition?

The superlative definition is: *that which is eaten to sustain life, provide energy, and promote the healing and repairing of tissues.*

Let's think about that.

Does a doughnut fit that definition?

Sure, a doughnut will give you energy, but it is not the kind of energy you want—a quick rush followed by a crash. You want a sustained and even supply of energy to propel you through the day.

Is a doughnut going to sustain life?

Sure, it will keep you alive, but it will not help you live the vibrant life you want to live.

Does a doughnut promote the healing and repair of tissues?

If garbage goes in, then garbage comes out. A doughnut will not provide the building blocks for high-quality tissue. It is absent of quality nutrients.

Your body is constantly mending tissues, building new cells, repairing old cells, and creating new hormones and brain chemicals that help you feel energized and invigorated. How do you think your body continually creates these things?

It uses the building blocks in your food. Every molecule in your body begins at the end of your fork, meaning your food provides the raw materials for your body to build new cells, generate healthy blood, balance hormones and neurotransmitters, and produce energy.

The microscopic biochemical machinery placing these building blocks together include enzymes, cofactors, and innumerable cell types. They require nutrients to operate; namely vitamins, minerals, fats, proteins, and carbohydrates, all of which you can find in your food. The body functions only as well as its complex and microscopic machinery can. That means you need enough of those nutrients in your diet every day so you can feel your best.

What Food Is and How It Should Be Used

In the previous chapter, we talked about how food is fuel for your body to repair tissues and perform at its optimum. For these reasons, think of your food as your medicine. A nutrient-dense diet can provide health, while a diet lacking in nutrients can take health away.

As Hippocrates is often credited with saying, "Let thy food be thy medicine."

Commonly, food is exclusively perceived as a source of pleasure, stress release, or just eating for the sake of eating. Do you understand? Many people rely on food for pleasure because they might not experience enough pleasure elsewhere in their life.

Food choices are frequently made as a reaction to stress. The foods chosen to manage stress tend not to be the healthiest. For example, junk food can provide a quick spike of pleasure that mediates stress in the moment, but often leaves you feeling worse later.

To dig out of this hole, switch your thinking to see food as fuel and medicine. Remember *an ounce of prevention is worth a pound of cure*, which emphasizes the power of prevention in staving off disease before it arises. You can try your best to cure your disease after it has developed. By then, you might already be taking medication to manage the condition, but even better would be to prevent it from occurring in the first place.

Maintaining health is an ongoing process in which our body is constantly changing, and food is one factor determining the ongoing result. Give your body what it needs, and it will achieve optimal health every day. The *side effect* of achieving health daily through nutrition is the prevention of chronic diseases like heart disease, diabetes, obesity, cancer, cardiovascular disease, osteoporosis, and Alzheimer's. This is very well documented by substantial research. (Centers for Disease Control and Prevention B; Ballarini et al. 2021; Muñoz-Garach, García-Fontana, and Muñoz-Torres 2020)

It certainly affects your mental-emotional well-being as well. If you are struggling with depression or anxiety, then fine-tuning your food choices will go a long way. You are making a choice every single day with the food you choose to put in your mouth about your health and about whether your health is getting better or worse. What you decide to buy at the store, cook at home, and put into your mouth are all choices you make.

What will you choose?

Epigenetics is the science of how your genetics change over time. It shows that choices you make every day transform the way your genes are expressed, which play a role in determining health. This means the decisions you make today not only affect *your* well-being but that of your offspring. Yes, that means your children and even your children's children. The everyday food choices you make are about more than just you.

Eating for Both Pleasure and Health

You might be thinking: *Sure, doc, this sounds great and all, but I want to enjoy what I eat!* Contrary to what most believe, you can do both.

As your body adapts to natural, whole foods, your taste buds actually change. In fact, they are always changing! The problem is they are bombarded with processed foods and artificial flavors engineered to make you crave more of these foods. Food production companies essentially want you addicted to their product because it is good for their business. If you give your body a break from the over-stimulation of foods and allow your body to readjust to whole foods, then you can enjoy the natural pleasure your body evolved to enjoy over thousands of years of evolution.

There are also many different recipes you can learn. With a little practice, you can create dishes that are not only delicious, but also beneficial for your health.

It takes commitment to your health and willingness to experiment. You would not be the first to reap the benefits of such changes with your nutrition—so many of our practice members have done just that. You will taste new flavors, like the natural sweetness of a carrot and all the complex flavors of a radish or raspberry. This is not about being 100 percent fixed on eating healthy foods or about avoiding other types of food. Instead, it is redefining your relationship with food and creating new habits.

You can eventually find balance in your approach to eating. You might be at a restaurant and occasionally have something you wouldn't normally have, and that's fine. Other foods become an occasional, voluntary indulgence rather than something you habitually rely on or a craving that you unwillingly give in to. The difference here is that you have strengthened your body through proper nutrition, so your health is much more robust and resilient if you deviate from time to time. Optimal health is about balance in the end. It is not about taking away your sources of pleasure; it is about expanding your ability to enjoy both your food and your life more completely.

HOW FOOD CAN FEED OR FIGHT DISEASE

Our health is always getting either better or worse; it is never staying the same. Food is foundational to your health, so it can either help or hurt you. It is a direct influence on whether your health is improving or worsening every day.

You can choose to eat foods not made to aid your health, supporting the companies that make them, or you can choose to consume foods provided by nature to support your health. The biochemical composition of food is either feeding disease or fighting it.

Processed Foods

Have you ever asked if a friend has any snacks in the house? Usually this is processed food, and it is such a big part of the American diet. Processed foods are essentially any food that has gone through processing of any kind, such as pasteurization. Packaged foods are often adulterated with preservatives to prolong their shelf-life, so it's also a good idea to avoid any food that comes sealed in a box, bag, or container. It does not come directly from nature, at least not without being altered in some way. Processing and packaging often damage the nutrient quality of food.

This low quality also manifests with genetic modification of foods, also called *genetically modified organisms* (GMOs). There are also pesticides in produce. Any food that is not organic exposes you to these pesticides, chemicals, and other toxins, burdening your body's toxic load.

These chemicals in our foods create inflammation in the body, so it is important for you to read nutrition labels and avoid anything that has a scary ingredient list with any words you have trouble pronouncing. One example is BHA, which stands for *butylated hydroxyanisole*. That word is the kind of scary and chemical-sounding name you do not want or need to have in your food. Foods with additives such as these are not created to support health—they are created to get you addicted, so you will continue buying them.

The companies that produce these foods are focused on business, marketing, and profit—*not* your health. The profit motive drives the production and sale of processed foods. Do not fall victim to it. Often these foods need synthetic vitamins and minerals added to them to prevent you from developing nutrient deficiencies.

Earlier I mentioned the importance of vitamins and minerals for enzymes, cells, and cofactors. These processed foods are usually lacking in nutrients, so companies add synthetic versions of vitamins. You might only think of nutrient deficiencies when you think of third-world countries, but these deficiencies absolutely create clinical problems and clinical diseases even in first-world countries like ours. The economics of food production are not in favor of your health, so you must be smarter than the system.

Whole Foods

Natural foods contain all the nutrients, vitamins, minerals, proteins, fats, and carbohydrates you need to thrive. Unprocessed foods have a rich concentration of these nutrients, and sometimes even an overabundance. Eating this way, your body is filled up to nutrient repletion and will discard the extra that it does not need.

This means eating as close to nature as possible and avoiding the foods stripped of nutrients. Focus on naturally grown foods, like grass-fed organic beef from a sustainable, ethical, local farm. *That* is eating directly from nature.

Think of a carrot you pull directly from the ground; there are thousands of biochemical nutrient compounds contained within—thousands working in synergy with vitamin A to achieve beneficial health results in your body. You need the whole symphony of nutrition in a single carrot, not the isolated components of vitamin A, because a supplement is missing all nutrient counterparts arriving with it in vegetable form.

Change Your Thinking!

Rather than shopping the whole grocery store, focus on the outside perimeter of the store. This is typically where most grocers stock whole foods: fresh fruits, vegetables, meats, and sometimes a bulk section with varieties of nuts, whole grains, and dried fruits. The center of the store is typically where packaged, processed foods are found: cereals, crackers, chips, canned meats and sauces, sugary beverages, and candy.

The guidelines for healthy eating are one half of the plate vegetables and the other half of the plate composed of proteins and fats. For example, you have a plate full of broccoli and radishes and the other half a full mixture of grass-fed beef with half an avocado. Protein is especially important; see the action item for this chapter for details.

Food Sensitivities and Inflammation (Symptoms and Conditions)

Many are familiar with peanut allergies. When someone touches or eats peanuts, it triggers an anaphylactic reaction. Their heart rate rises, they become red and swollen, and they have trouble breathing. That is a food allergy. Now contrast that with a food sensitivity. Unlike a food allergy, an immediate reaction, a food sensitivity reaction is delayed over hours or days. When you eat a food, even healthy foods like eggs, salmon, or almonds, your body may have a negative reaction that develops gradually. The problem here is that you may not realize it because the reaction happens so slowly and can affect body systems other than just your stomach and intestines.

It can cause acne on the skin, abdominal discomfort, bloating, pain, and issues with bowel movements in the gastrointestinal system, and even cause brain fog. This is happening because the reaction is creating inflammation not only in your intestines, but also systemically. This systemic effect occurs because these foods create a condition called *leaky gut syndrome*, also called *intestinal hyperpermeability*.

Your intestines, which are essentially a long tube starting at the bottom of the stomach and ending at the anus, filter microscopic particles of nutrients to be absorbed into your bloodstream. If the small intestines are not functioning well, damage to that filtration action can cause it to become more permeable than it should be. Larger, undigested food particles can then pass through the intestinal walls. This leads to issues elsewhere in the body, such as autoimmune disease, because your immune system reacts to the particles as invaders and a potential threat. Your immune system becomes dysregulated and reacts to the new food particles in the bloodstream, producing inflammation and other complications.

Nutrient deficiencies are another factor that can affect different organ systems. When you are not feeding your body enough micronutrients, your health suffers. *Essential fatty acids* are called *essential* because your body cannot make them from scratch. This is compared to other types of fats your body can produce on its own, but it cannot produce the essential fatty acids like omega-3s—we must get these directly from food.

Omega-3 fatty acids are part of every cell membrane in the body, which help maximize nerve cell function, hormone production, and regulation of inflammation. You can get omega-3s in fish and nuts, flaxseed oil, and certain dark green, leafy vegetables. Insufficient essential fatty acids create dry, scaly skin; brittle, cracking nails; and acne. If deficient throughout your lifetime, you are also much more likely to develop cognitive decline and Alzheimer's (Thomas et al. 2015; Cole, Ma, and Frautschy 2009).

Calcium is important for building strong bones, as well as important for nerve function, muscle function, and heart health. If you are not getting adequate intake of calcium-rich foods in your diet, or if you are not absorbing your calcium due to poor gut health or lack of dietary vitamin D—which helps absorb calcium—then that leaves you at a higher risk for developing osteoporosis and potential fractures. You can also develop numbness and tingling in your extremities or muscle cramps. You want to increase your sources of calcium in your diet but also eliminate possible substances preventing the absorption of calcium, like caffeine and alcohol.

Omega-3 fats and calcium are just two examples of common nutrient deficiencies. There are many more.

THE IMPORTANCE OF INDIVIDUALIZING NUTRITION

We must figure out the right diet for you. There is no one-size-fits-all diet. Most people believe when they fail diets and don't stick to one, it is their fault. They are disappointed and discouraged they did not see the benefits they expected.

When people do not stick with diets and do not get the results they want, it is also because the diet is not made for them. It is not created in a way that it is going to be sustainable for them as a unique individual. The best diet for you is not going to be the best diet for your sister, mom, boss, or friend. It is unique to you, so if we are going to get you unstuck and get you on the path to optimal health, we need to find the best diet for you specifically.

One Diet Does Not Fit All

There are no cookie-cutter diets that will work for everyone. However, there are common themes to a healthy diet. There are general overarching principles which we have discussed already, but there is more to that story.

One aspect we have previously discussed is figuring out what your unique food sensitivities are. What foods are creating issues for you—specifically which foods are creating unnecessary inflammation and inhibiting your body from achieving full health?

Another aspect is that certain dietary patterns may or may not be appropriate for different medical conditions. For example, if you have a thyroid condition, we want you to avoid certain food compounds, specifically *goitrogens*. Goitrogens are molecular compounds in raw brassica vegetables, such as Brussels sprouts, broccoli, and cauliflower, that interfere with thyroid function. If you already have a thyroid condition, these raw vegetables will generally need to be avoided. That is one example of how we individualize medical nutrition to you as a unique person.

Another factor we want to take into consideration is medication use because medications waste nutrients, causing the body to eliminate certain nutrients your body actually needs. This is another way nutrient deficiencies can develop.

Common examples are statin drugs for high cholesterol, which waste CoQ10 in the body. It is important to at least supplement with CoQ10 if you are taking a statin, and then over the long term, the goal is to use nutrition and other foundations to help you decrease the need for a statin. These are all important elements that need to be accounted for when developing a treatment and lifestyle plan for you.

Using an Elimination Diet

An elimination diet is when we eliminate certain foods from your diet. This is how we identify and remove foods that are obstacles to your healing. We want to eliminate the foods that are suppressing your body's ability to heal and function optimally.

How do we figure which foods are to be avoided?

First, we need to remove foods from your diet most commonly found to be an issue for people in general and second, remove foods that are often culprits behind the symptoms you are experiencing. Then we pay attention to what changes in your health. That could be anything from your sleep quality to your mood and digestive issues. If these issues go away, then we know there is a correlation with the food you have removed.

You remove the food for four to twelve weeks, because that's the time it takes your body to fully clear its immune reaction—in the form of antibodies—to the foods. This process requires patience. Once the elimination phase is complete, the *reintroduction phase* begins. This is when we choose one food at a time to reintroduce into your diet. We observe whether there are any adverse effects when you return to eating that food. If there is a reaction, we've confirmed that food causes issues for you and should continue to be avoided.

Let us say you eliminated eggs and noticed your acne decreases. Then you add eggs back into your diet and see acne symptoms returning. As a result, you now know that eggs are likely creating a negative reaction in your body.

Next, you will remove that food for a longer period to allow your body time to heal. That does not mean you will not be able to eat eggs ever again, but your body needs the opportunity to heal without the offending foods before you may be able to eat them again.

Positive Effects

When you decide to make changes to your diet and with your habits about nutrition, you can see immense leaps in health. Taking this step on its own can change your life. It is not uncommon, and rather expected, to see improvements in energy, mood, and stability. Your appearance of health, your vibrancy, and your shedding weight are healthy side effects of establishing optimal health. You may notice after undertaking this process of eliminating problem foods from the diet, you look and feel vibrant and almost glowing. That kind of effect can be expected in addition to all the smaller benefits.

For the first time, you can lower your medication use because your doctor no longer sees the need for it. The doctor may see your blood pressure coming down or weight decreasing, and when they see their patient's symptoms decreasing, they say, *well, there is no more need for you to be taking this much medication.*

Naturally the prescribing doctor chooses to lower the dose or remove it completely from your care plan. These specific effects may or may not happen for you, but these types of positive changes are bound to happen when you decide to elevate your diet.

Action Item

- *Eat protein-rich foods. They control food motivation centers in the brain to decrease the tendency to overeat throughout the remainder of the day* (Weigle et al. 2005; Blom et al. 2006). *Eat 25 to 30 grams of protein for every single meal, especially for breakfast. This is the equivalent of about four eggs or a piece of meat about the size of your palm. This one change alone stimulates fat loss. Don't be surprised to see an initial loss of ten pounds in the first month.*

- *The guidelines we recommend for healthy eating are filling one-half of your plate with vegetables and the other half of the plate with proteins and fats. For example, you have a plate full of broccoli and radishes and on the other half a full mixture of grass-fed beef with half an avocado.*

CHAPTER FOUR

The Importance of Energy

SLEEP

Energy is a broad term, referring to the essence of life flowing through all living things. The presence of energy is the difference between something alive and something dead. It is a biological necessity. Every cell in your body needs enough energy to work together with all other cells to create life. This is what creates vital functions, such as your heartbeat, brainwaves, blood circulation, breathing—everything necessary for you to maintain life.

Since ancient times, the practitioners of Chinese medicine have called this energy *Qi*, while the practitioners of Ayurvedic medicine have called it *Prana*. Practitioners long ago used the information they had at their disposal, without the advantages of modern science. To our way of thinking, this understanding was forcibly more limited and abstract. With the advent of modern technology, however, science has discovered a biochemical, microscopic basis for this energy in every single cell of your body, called *adenosine triphosphate* (ATP).

ATP molecules are organic molecular compounds that provide energy to living cells to perform their function. This all means our health and healing depend on approaching our lifestyle and wellness in a way that supports the balance of energy.

When we say *energy regulation*, we are talking about the way your body creates, uses, and replenishes energy. You want to have more than enough energy to get up in the morning and propel yourself through the day, and an appropriately lesser amount of energy in the evening, so you can fall asleep and regenerate energy again for the next day.

There are three main processes at large that regulate our energy:

1. Sleep
2. Stress
3. Fitness

There is an incredibly strong link between sleep and your health. Sleep is the time when your body recuperates and replenishes the energy it needs to keep your heart beating, your lungs breathing, and your muscles working. Your body uses energy to generate feelings of pleasure or peace, fear or stress, and all the thoughts you have. These depend on the flow of energy, and sleep is the first determining factor of your energy flow.

Ongoing lack of sleep can be a huge detractor from health. It makes you feel tired and frustrated. It impacts your mental and physical performance and your body's ability to function. If you are sleeping well consistently, and then sleep poorly for one night, that is no big deal; you will bounce back quickly. The cumulative effect of losing sleep over weeks, months, or years is linked to development of chronic disease, putting yourself at risk for reduced immunity, decreased brain function, cardiovascular disease, and more. You must get a handle on sleep, so your health can be the best it can be.

The Physiology and Activity of Sleep

Underlying the process of sleep are patterns of brain activity and energy regulation that your body goes through every night. There are different phases to a full night's sleep.

First, as the day ends in the evening, your brain activity slows down.

Once the sun sets, the absence of light eventually stimulates the release of melatonin from your brain, a sleep-inducing hormone that tones down your brain activity, so you start feeling sleepy.

Once you are finally asleep, you enter natural cycles of brain activity divided into the two phases of sleep:

1. Non-REM Sleep

   This is when deep sleep occurs—that is, sleep that is generally harder to wake up from. Your heart rate and your brain activity slow. Your body repairs and builds bones and muscle tissue. Your immune system is strengthened.

2. REM sleep

   REM stands for *rapid eye movement*. Dreaming occurs in this phase. During REM sleep you have increased brain activity, muscle relaxation, and vivid dreams. This is when your brain processes the events of the day, so better learning and long-term memory can take place. Feel-good hormones, such as *dopamine* and *serotonin*, are produced to help boost your mood and give you energy.

If you are not getting REM sleep, your body is not going to have those hormones to keep you feeling good. As a result, you might struggle with lower mood and negative thoughts and feelings. REM sleep does not happen until about an hour to an hour and a half after falling asleep. Your body is constantly cycling between non-REM and REM sleep. One full cycle between both phases takes about one and a half to two hours total.

With aging, we begin to see more sleeping issues, which usually means less non-REM sleep. Naturally, as you age, your body gets less non-REM sleep, and you will sleep less. Considering that you will start missing out on more of that precious non-REM sleep you were getting when you were younger, we want to maximize your sleep as much as possible. Whether you are having issues falling asleep or staying asleep, we must figure out which part of sleep is problematic to determine how to correct it.

Causes and Effects of Poor Sleep

When people have trouble sleeping, it is either due to difficulty falling asleep or with trouble staying asleep. These problems are not one and the same because they are due to different causes.

Most people know what it feels like to not sleep well and feel sleep deprived. You wake up and feel groggy and unable to focus. At its worst, sleep deprivation can make you feel like you got hit by a truck. You have a short temper, your moods are more volatile, and you are not able to make the best decisions. Worst of all, you are dragging because your energy is diminished.

Poor decision-making and impaired reaction time can make driving more dangerous because your hands, feet, and brain are not working as quickly as they should be.

Inability to sleep is a symptom—a sign there is something deeper going on. There are many complications of long-term sleep issues you want to avoid. We have already named a few related to concentration, memory, and mood. The list continues:

- Diabetes (Knutson 2006; Mullington et al. 2010)

- Cardiovascular disease (Kasasbeh, Chi, Krishnaswamy 2006; Ruesten et al. 2012)

- Obesity (Taheri 2006; Mullington et al. 2010)

- Depression (Zimmerman et al. 2006)

- Alzheimer's (Shokri-Kojori et al. 2018; Ma et al. 2020)

- Cancer (Ruesten et al. 2012)

Additionally, there's a higher risk of all-cause mortality—death from any cause (Mullington et al. 2010).

Is there anything it doesn't cause? *Yikes!*

Any combination of these health detriments can develop over time if we are not sleeping well. If you currently have any of those conditions, or if you have anxiety or high stress, depression or mood swings, thyroid or cardiovascular disease or diabetes, poor sleep is a contributor to that.

Sleep gives your heart and cardiovascular system a needed rest, especially during the non-REM phase. So if you are missing out on non-REM sleep then you are more likely to develop health issues such as:

- Cardiovascular disease
- Cancer
- Strokes
- Heart attack (Ruesten et al. 2012)
- Diabetes (Ruesten et al. 2012)
- High blood pressure
- Congestive heart failure (Javaheri, Javaheri, and Javaheri 2013)

A lack of sleep also contributes to high levels of blood proteins, such as C-reactive protein (CRP), which is the most important marker of inflammation in the body (Mullington et al. 2010). It is a good idea to test for CRP. Elevated levels can be followed by hardening of the arteries, resulting in atherosclerosis.

Lack of sleep also triggers your body to release more adrenaline or cortisol during the day. This high level of stress hormones will only make symptoms worse, regardless of what they are. For example, your blood pressure will remain high, and your heart will be unable to recuperate overnight. Your hormones suffer, including leptin and ghrelin. Remember, *leptin* is the appetite suppressor and *ghrelin* is the appetite stimulant. With sleep issues these hormones are imbalanced, namely low levels of leptin and high ghrelin (Taheri et al. 2004).

That means you are more likely to overeat, taking in more calories and more carbohydrates, and therefore are more likely to be overweight. There is also a growth hormone which boosts muscle mass, repairs cells and tissues, and burns fat, so without good sleep you will not be repairing your tissues very well. Sex hormones like testosterone and estrogen also burn fat and support fertility. You might develop trouble conceiving or have issues burning fat and optimizing body weight or muscle mass, so poor sleep will certainly not help optimize your physique.

Energy can suffer as well. Your blood sugar rises and falls during sleep. Your insulin, a hormone controlling your blood sugar, can be affected by a week of decreased sleep. This means your blood sugar levels can resemble that of a person with diabetes. It also means higher risks of developing diabetes over time.

The last element is immune function, which prevents you from getting sick and helps you heal fast if you do get sick. Know what to expect if your immune system becomes compromised.

Now that you understand the effects of poor sleep, ask yourself: *What causes poor sleep?*

Stress is one major cause, whether it is your work, your marriage, or your never–ending to–do list, tension from the stress of life can prevent your brain from shutting down completely and attaining a good night's rest.

Mood issues like anxiety and depression can also throw off your brain rhythms. There is such a thing as too much sleep. Rather than sleeping too little, depression can cause you to sleep too much, to be in bed for twelve or more hours at a time. You want everything in balance—the Goldilocks Principle—even the amount of sleep you get.

Pain due to physical ailments or medical conditions, such as acid reflux, heart disease, or chronic musculoskeletal pain, can keep you awake at night.

Pharmaceuticals such as high blood pressure medication can even contribute to sleep difficulty.

Lifestyle choices are the last and most important factors. These are the activities you engage in every day. Some examples include:

- Bright light exposure before bed, typically from your TV or phone

- Watching your favorite show while lying in your bed

- Eating or exercising within a couple of hours before bedtime

- Consuming alcohol, sugar, or caffeine four to five hours before bed, or for some people, at any time during the day

- Failing to exercise during the day

- Failure to adequately manage your stress

- Not having a nightly pre-bedtime routine

The good thing is that you have direct control over each of these and can make changes to them as soon as you decide to do so.

Causes and Effects of Great Sleep

Now that we talked about the effects of poor sleep, let's talk about the benefits of great-quality sleep. Sleep restores you physically, mentally, and even emotionally. It plays a big role in your immune system, metabolism, mood, memory, and more. It is crucial to give your brain, muscles, and organs a much-needed break so they can do their job. This usually means about eight hours of sleep per night for a young adult.

If you feel refreshed, energetic, and alert from morning to evening, then you probably received enough sleep the night before. Because of this, your energy, mood, and mental clarity remain stable throughout the day. Your ability to manage and recover from stress determines your resilience. These effects are much the opposite of poor sleep.

If you are not feeling alert throughout the day, then you need to figure out the cause, so you do not rely on stimulants like coffee to get you through the day. Good sleep decreases your risk for developing chronic disease, such as cardiovascular disease and cancer, because you have fewer stress hormones flowing through your body during the day.

Your heart, vascular system, and the rest of your body are receiving frequent opportunities to heal without exposure to stress hormones. You have enhanced immune function, so you will have a larger immune capacity to fight off common infections and be less likely to develop other chronic diseases or immune deficiencies.

Your appetite hormones, leptin and ghrelin, are more balanced, so your appetite is in check. Your body's ability to burn fat and build muscle is improved because growth hormones, testosterone, and estrogen are optimized.

If you rely on over-the-counter sleep medications, then try the following changes. To nobody's surprise, the causes of great sleep are essentially the opposite of habits that create poor sleep. But let's clarify them anyway:

- Develop a regular pre–bedtime routine.

- Eat nutritious meals full of nutrient-dense foods during the day.

- Do not eat two hours before bed.

- Avoid alcohol, sugar, and caffeine.

- Avoid smoking.

- Manage your stress as best as you can, relaxing before bed.

- Take time to unwind to help smooth out and calm brain activity.

- Keep your bedroom environment dark, quiet, and sleep friendly.

- Get sunlight and exercise during the day to help recharge your energy and regulate your brain rhythm to promote good sleep at night.

- Avoid electronics and bright screens like TV and phone. Do so for at least sixty minutes before bedtime.

All of these will help maximize sleep, so you can look good, feel good, and live freely.

STRESS

Stress, like sleep, has a significant influence on both your mind and body. Usually when you think of stress, you think of *bad* stress, but as you will see, there is both good and bad stress, and both are contributors to your well-being.

Good Stress

Stress, in general, is a response. It is a response to any influence that causes you to adapt, whether that force is physical stress, like manual labor or exercise, or mental stress, from making decisions at work or paying attention to driving in severe weather.

Either way, your body and mind adapt to the stress by growing and strengthening. Some of it is *good*, meaning it causes a healthy response that makes you stronger. It provides the stimulus needed for growth and strengthening.

This is what we call *eustress*; the prefix *eu-* is Greek for *good*. The clearest example of this is exercise—like weightlifting—which is putting a physical load on your body. This actually breaks down muscle tissue in the short term.

Then what happens?

The body responds to the stressful event by building stronger muscle fibers over time. This is your body's intelligent way of preparing to encounter that stress again. Those muscle fibers were damaged, and the body repairs them by becoming stronger than they were before the exercise.

This also occurs within your immune system as it learns to defend you from exposure to microbes—viruses, bacteria, filth, soil, and so on. Exposure mildly stresses the immune system, which prompts its defensive action against that particular threat. The result is you develop immunity to the virus or bacteria.

The same happens mentally and emotionally, and this is how to keep your cognition strong: by engaging in activities that get your cognitive and emotional energy flowing. Maybe you have an intellectually demanding job, or you are a student, or your primary relationship is emotionally challenging. Your brain and your cognition respond to those stressful stimuli by becoming stronger—as long as the stress does not persist for too long without giving your body a chance to heal. Like your muscle fibers and exercise, your body and mind need a break from the stress regularly to give them a chance to rest.

While we may have heard stress is bad, the main points to remember are:

- We *need* stress.

- Not all stress is bad.

- Some stress is necessary for achieving optimal health.

Bad Stress and Inflammation

We've previously described how a low level of stress that persists over a long period of time can be harmful, but also noted that stress can be harmful when encountered in higher intensity within a more condensed length of time. For example, consider the stress of a car crash compared with physical exercise.

Low-grade stress applied over the long term without giving your body a break can also cause harm. For example, pain can develop in the wrist from the repetitive movements of typing on a computer keyboard.

There is a saying: *The dose makes the poison.* For example, drinking too much water can kill you. It is not that the substance itself determines whether something is good or bad; is the quantity of it or the duration of exposure to it.

Stressors on your body include:

- Toxins in the environment

- Chronic exposure to microbes

- Chronic infections

- Excessive exercising—running a hundred miles rather than five may do more harm than good

- Extreme or persistent emotional states at work, home, etc.

We need everything in moderation. This physiologically affects your hormone balance. Cortisol, the stress hormone, causes activation of both the fight-or-flight response and your immune system. The immune system is activated when we have too much stress or the stress persists. That chronic activation from the stress response leads to chronic inflammation, so inflammation runs rampant for too long.

This leads to imbalance all over the body, such as:

- Gut problems

- Mood problems

- Brain-related issues with focus, cognition, mood, and energy

- Hormonal imbalance

- Inability to lose weight and burn fat

With people who have inflammatory issues and conditions, it is essential to discover the causes of stress in their life so they can be addressed.

Stress Reduction

The good news about this bad stress is that you have more control over it than you think.

The first step is to identify the sources of stress in your life, whether it's work, your personal relationships, low-quality or reactive foods in your diet, or not enough exercise. Fat tissue in the body creates oxidative stress that furthers inflammation in your body. Instead, you want to rebalance and take control of your lifestyle to set you and your health up for maximum success. This means optimizing your diet, enhancing sleep, and looking at stress reduction practices like meditation to find something that works for you.

There are multiple forms of meditation for stress reduction. There are movement meditation practices like Qi Gong and Tai Chi. There are more exercise-related methods, such as yoga or conventional exercise, like running or weight training. These are within your control, and it is important to discover what is sustainable and maximally effective for you and your unique lifestyle preferences.

FITNESS

Exercise is obviously important for optimal health. Maybe you are someone who exercised in the past but have fallen out of the habit. Maybe you are doing exercise now but still haven't reached your health goals, and you see exercise working for everyone else but you. Perhaps you do not have the energy to start exercising; you don't feel well and simply can't get yourself to do it. Whichever of these apply to you, first working on all the other Pillars will set your body up for feeling well enough to start a fitness routine and to find results where you were previously stuck.

Effects of Exercise on Circulation, Stress, and Inflammation

The effects of exercise are almost infinite. Exercise is beneficial to nearly every organ system in your body. It regulates the nervous system so you can sleep well at night, feel calm, obtain mood stability, and manage stress. It also sharpens your ability to focus and think clearly and effectively.

Then, of course, there is what I like to call *body re-composition*. This idea of body re-composition is not limited to only burning fat or building muscle. Instead, we want to do both simultaneously. That way you'll not only feel great, but also achieve that lean, toned, and healthy-looking physique. Remember how your muscle fibers undergo damage and become stronger in turn? Exercise concurrently decreases fat and increases muscle. But that's not all.

Exercise positively impacts blood flow and circulatory power for two reasons:

1. The heart pumps harder, and the blood vessels open to allow more blood flow.

2. Your muscles naturally pump the blood in your vessels by way of *muscle contracture*—the contraction of muscles pushes the blood along.

This increased blood flow, if produced regularly, improves cardiovascular disease and other vascular issues like cold hands and feet, and reduces risk for strokes, heart attacks, and diabetes.

Fat tissue is generally inflammatory and muscle tissue is anti-inflammatory, so the more body re-composition we achieve by optimizing the ratio of muscle tissue to fat tissue, the more anti-inflammatory power your body will have. This also applies to the brain—balancing neurotransmitters and decreasing inflammation in the brain to make you feel good—making exercise a natural antidepressant.

Types of Exercise

There are basically three types of exercise.

1. Everyday movement

   Exercise does not need to mean going to the gym to sweat like crazy and work super hard. You are exercising throughout your day when you're engaged in tasks such as simply walking around, carrying the laundry, hauling groceries from the store, and gardening. These activities get your body moving to keep your joints and muscles loose, supple, and strong. Keep on moving for good circulation!

2. Cardio

   Cardiometabolic activity is what most people do at the gym when running or biking, for example. Cardio activities are important because they provide the health benefits just discussed. But they are not usually going to give you the most bang for your buck in terms of achieving the desired benefits of body re-composition, hormonal optimization, energy, focus, and sleep. A lot of people try to spend an hour and a half on the treadmill every day, but most quit because they are not getting results, and frankly, it is boring.

3. Resistance Exercise

   Higher intensity in nature, *resistance exercise* puts your body under higher physical stress loads for a short period. This could be achieved through *high-intensity interval training* (HIIT) intervals of twenty to sixty seconds of rapid, high-intensity activities—such as weightlifting, calisthenics, or running—alternating with short periods of rest. Both HIIT and weight training rev your metabolism more effectively, creating a good stress in your body. They stimulate your body to burn more fat and build more muscle.

Speaking of burning fat, you also experience what is called the *after-burn effect*. The after-burn effect means your body will continue burning fat throughout the rest of the day, even when you are sitting on the couch or making dinner. This is not true for regular cardio exercise or other types of lower-intensity movement, in which benefits are only achieved during the exercise session.

All health benefits of anti-inflammation, mood support, cognitive sharpening, blood flow, fat burning, and muscle building are much more potent with resistance exercise. It also requires less time while giving you more bang for your buck. But regardless of which type you choose, always prioritize safety by learning proper technique to minimize risk of injury.

An Individualized Program

Exercise is not one–size–fits–all. There are general principles, such as those I've already discussed, but additionally, you need to support your goals in the ways most likely to achieve health independence for the rest of your life. You need habits, like exercise, that you are going to stick with.

You need to find what works for you and your lifestyle, something enjoyable. Your unique medical situation also needs to be considered. That is why it is important to work with a medical professional who can help recommend types of exercise to best fit your unique circumstance to maximize safety and efficacy. Individualizing your plan will make it as effective, safe, and sustainable as needed.

Action Item

Sleep

- *Avoid exposure to light and digital screens one hour before bed—phones, TV, computer, bright lamps.*

- *Create an environment conducive to sleep—one that is calm, quiet, dimly lit, with minimal stimulus.*

Stress

- *Start a 5-minute daily mindfulness practice. This will increase your resilience to emotional stress for the rest of the day and maximize your focus and productivity.*

- *How do you meditate? It is simple; sit in a quiet room and be present. Use a guided meditation if you'd like; many free guided meditations can be found on the internet.*

- *Do this every morning upon waking, before you eat your high-protein breakfast. Increase your session by five minutes every ten days.*

Fitness

- *Walk briskly at least once daily*

- *If your fitness capacity is low, begin with ten minutes daily. Walk outside, choose a landmark to reach in five minutes, then walk back.*

- *If you have intermediate capacity, begin with thirty minutes and add intervals of jogging or speed-walking until you feel your heart rate increase, then slow down to a brisk walk again. Complete ten intervals within the thirty-minute time block.*

CHAPTER FIVE

The Importance of Hormones

THYROID

There are three main groups of hormones affecting our overall health. The first group is thyroid hormones. Thyroid disease affects many people today, primarily *hypo*-thyroidism, which means the thyroid gland is under-functioning. We will also discuss *hyper*-thyroidism, which is when the gland is over-functioning. Hypothyroidism is the most common form of thyroid disease, and women are affected five times more often than men (Garber et al. 2012).

Most people know of a type of autoimmune hypothyroid called *Hashimoto's disease*. Since inflammation plays a role in thyroid dysfunction, the medical term for it is *chronic lymphocytic thyroiditis*. The suffix *-itis* in medical lingo refers to the presence of inflammation. The thyroid gland is inflamed, but why? Ninety percent of hypothyroidism is due to an autoimmune process (Amino 1988). Thus, if you have hypothyroid, make sure your thyroid antibody levels are checked as it is possible you actually have Hashimoto's.

Your Time to Thrive

There are antithyroid antibodies present contributing to the inflammation. This means that you must treat more than just the thyroid; the immune system also needs to be addressed. This requires proper evaluation and testing, which we talk about later in the chapter, and it also means addressing the Pillars of Health discussed throughout the book. The good news is that this condition often improves substantially with this approach, a functional evaluation in conjunction with lifestyle management and holistic therapies.

Hyperthyroidism means excessive functioning of the thyroid gland. When autoimmune in nature, it is referred to as *Graves' disease*. This condition is triggered by autoimmune antibodies overstimulating the thyroid gland. Traditional treatment is medication or surgery to remove the thyroid. However, surgically removing it is a final resort—a drastic measure that technically reverses the condition.

The consequence of removal is hypothyroidism. This makes sense because without a thyroid gland, the body is left with minimal to no thyroid function. This means you must take thyroid replacement medication for life. Knowing this, do everything you can to address your condition before that needs to happen.

Autoimmune conditions like thyroid disease typically cannot be cured, but remission to decrease the severity of symptoms and be able to live more freely is most certainly possible.

What Does the Thyroid Do?

The thyroid is a butterfly-shaped organ in the neck. It controls the release of thyroid hormones that control metabolism and energy use for every single cell in your body. Every cell in your body requires energy to perform its unique function, so thyroid hormones help keep your entire body working correctly.

However, the thyroid does not act on its own. The brain releases a hormone called TSH, which stands for *thyroid stimulating hormone.* You may be familiar with TSH because it is the most frequent marker tested when your doctor orders a blood test related to thyroid. Once released from the pituitary gland—a structure in the center of the brain— TSH stimulates the thyroid gland in your neck to release two hormones.

That is why it is called thyroid *stimulating* hormone, because it stimulates the thyroid to release T3 and T4, which ultimately influence nearly every cell in your body. T3 is the main hormone that does most of that work. T4 is a reserve pool of inactive hormone that your body must convert to T3 in order to use.

Think of it as the difference between crude oil and gasoline. T4 is like crude oil, in that processing is needed before your car can use it as fuel. T4 is converted into T3, the more active hormone, as needed. T3 is like gasoline that your car can easily use as fuel to produce energy.

Where does this conversion from T4 into T3 happen?

It happens both in the liver and digestive system. Normally, as T3 hormones (gasoline) are used by your body, the thyroid creates replacement T3 hormones as needed from the reserve pool of T4 (crude oil). But in hypothyroidism, your thyroid has less ability to do that. In addition to your thyroid's inability to produce enough T4, due to an autoimmune process attacking the thyroid gland itself, your body is commonly also unable to convert that T4 into active T3 due to dysfunction in the liver and the digestive system. That is why your body becomes deficient in thyroid hormone over time, and you feel tired, depressed, lethargic, and overweight. The conventional treatment is thyroid replacement medication. It is often effective in normalizing your TSH value on a blood test, but frequently fails to help you truly feel better.

Thyroid system

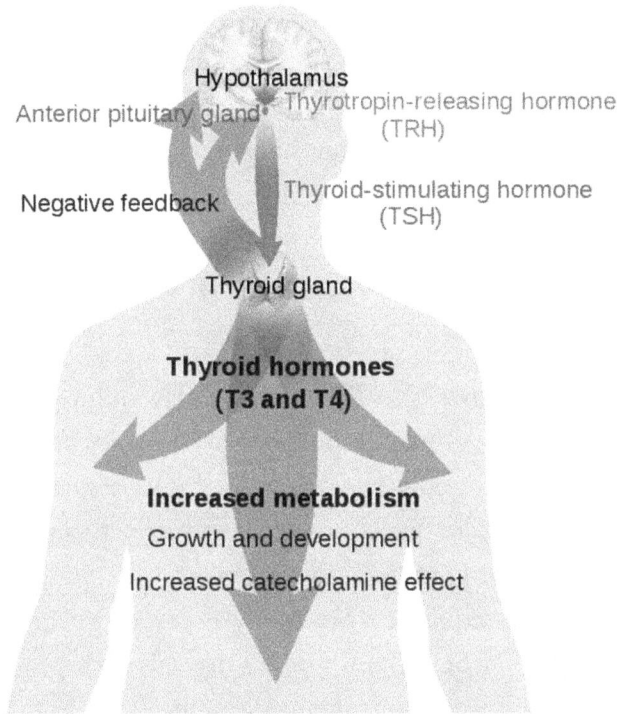

Hypothalamus

Anterior pituitary gland — Thyrotropin-releasing hormone (TRH)

Negative feedback

Thyroid-stimulating hormone (TSH)

Thyroid gland

Thyroid hormones (T3 and T4)

Increased metabolism

Growth and development

Increased catecholamine effect

en.wikipedia.org/wiki/Thyroid_hormones

Thyroid hormones influence many different organ systems (Shahid, Ashraf, and Sharma 2022). First, they largely affect your overall metabolism, which is the way your body turns food into energy and the way every one of your cells uses that energy. It is the way calories in your food are used, a large factor in determining whether weight will be lost or gained and whether your body will burn fat, *lipolysis*, or store fat, *lipogenesis.* When your thyroid works properly, it creates the right number of hormones to maintain your metabolism.

The thyroid also keeps the neurotransmitters in your brain and nervous system humming along for good mood and sharp thinking. It maintains your body temperature, heart rate, and cholesterol levels. Since it regulates the sex hormones testosterone and estrogen, strong fertility in men and women and healthy menstruation and ovulation cycles in women depend on thyroid function.

Thyroid hormones also direct the replacement of old cells with new ones—most importantly your skin and bones— to create vibrant-looking skin and build strong bones in the prevention of osteoporosis. The effect on digestion is incredibly important since it governs the production of stomach acid required to properly break down and absorb food. It also pushes it through the digestive tract for regular and healthy bowel movements. Finally, little known is its effect on many different elements of the immune system. So, ensuring proper immune function and resilience to inflammation, infection, and immune deficiency means firming up thyroid and hormone health (Jara et al. 2017).

Common Symptoms of Thyroid Disorder and Benefits of Correction

A person with hypothyroidism typically presents with these observable symptoms:

- Excess weight
- Dry skin and coarse hair
- Some hair loss
- Exhaustion

A person with hypothyroidism typically experiences symptoms such as:

- Fatigue
- Lack of energy sufficient to walk up stairs
- Depression
- Anxiety
- Forgetfulness or brain fog
- Constipation or other digestive issues
- Heavy or frequent menstruation
- Intolerance to cold temperatures
- Body temperature dysregulation

When the imbalance is corrected, massive changes can be seen in this picture. We see a person who appears leaner and more fit because they are burning fat and building toned muscle. The skin and hair are more vibrant and supple. They feel more energetic. They can go up and down the steps with no problem and do the things they want to do. Mood is improved and remains stable. Bowel movements are regular and easy. Cognition is clear with no more brain fog. The menstrual cycles are balanced and regular. Body temperature is steady. These are the shifts that are likely to occur for a person addressing their hypothyroid issues.

A person with hyperthyroidism presents as the opposite of a person with hypothyroidism, as these two conditions wreak havoc in your body in exactly opposite ways. Remember that someone with hyperthyroidism produces *too much* thyroid hormone. While hypothyroid slows and depresses the body's function, hyperthyroid speeds up and increases the body's function.

In a condition of hyperthyroidism, the following symptoms may occur:

- Organs are overstimulated—including the brain and nervous system—which leads the person to feel more anxious and irritable

- More nervous energy

- Sleeping trouble

- Tremor, or a fine trembling in the hand or fingers

- Increased heart rate and cholesterol levels

- Tendency to *run warm*, with increased sensitivity to heat, causing more sweat and feeling clammy more often

- Protruding eyes or eyes that appear enlarged

- Underweight, or metabolism burning too much energy; unintentional weight loss persists despite average appetite and food intake

- Changes in menstrual patterns

- Changes in bowel patterns, especially more loose or frequent bowels

- Thinner skin and fine, brittle hair

When the hyperthyroid imbalance is corrected, people finally appear more fit and well-toned. The hair and skin are fuller and more vibrant. Their mood is more relaxed overall and stable. They are not anxious or sweating all the time. Their body temperature is more consistently even, so they sleep better. They have less anxiety and irritability. Also, they have fewer palpitations and a more stable heart rate. Menstrual cycles are regular.

And finally, if you have hyperthyroid symptoms, they can alternate with hypothyroid symptoms. If you get treated for the hyperthyroidism, then you could switch into a hypothyroid state. Some people who have Hashimoto's might also have both hyperthyroid and hypothyroid symptoms. So, this can be confusing for patients, and even for healthcare providers, but requesting the appropriate testing can make all the difference in these cases.

You may have followed a doctor's recommendation to take thyroid medication for thyroid replacement. Three months later, the doctor may retest you and inform you your thyroid results are all normal, even though you still do not feel normal. Perhaps the doctor thinks the problem has been fixed, but you don't feel like you know you should be feeling. Or maybe you have not been prescribed medication, but the thyroid test results still come back normal, so the doctor has nothing to offer you.

There are two problems with the conventional protocol for evaluation and testing.

1. The first is that they run basic tests, enough to make sure there is no serious and life-threatening disease going on, to help you continue to survive, but not thrive. For testing, they will typically test markers limited to TSH and maybe T4. That is not going to cut it. You need more precise testing than that.

2. The second problem is that they use conventional reference ranges for interpreting the results. Conventional reference ranges are determined based on an average population, and you already know the average population is not a healthy population. Instead, it is better to use functional reference ranges, which determine their normal ranges based on a healthy population of people.

When you give a functional doctor your thyroid results, we interpret the same results in a different way—a functional interpretation. A *normal* TSH level to a conventional doctor is not necessarily going to be *normal* to a functional doctor. In this case, we might find what we call a *subclinical* hypothyroidism. Subclinical means that the result is not *abnormal* by the conventional perspective, but it is *subnormal* by a more functional perspective. This means we have found a potential cause for your suffering that we can treat, whereas otherwise, that may not have been the case.

Aside from hyperthyroidism and hypothyroidism, there are many other forms of thyroid diseases:

- *Primary hypothyroidism*, the problem being the actual thyroid gland itself.

- *Hypopituitarism*, the dysfunction of the pituitary gland in the brain, in which it is incorrectly sending TSH signals to the thyroid gland.

- *Thyroid under conversion*, when the liver or digestive system is not adequately converting T4 to T3. We see this with people who have gut and digestive problems, so we must address gut health as well.

- *Thyroid resistance*, in which all the cells in your body develop resistance to T3. This commonly happens when someone is on thyroid medicine for a long time and their body becomes resistant to it.

- *Autoimmune thyroid.* An example of this is Hashimoto's thyroiditis, which we discussed earlier. This is a state in which the immune system is activated against your thyroid gland.

To consider all possibilities and find the true cause of your symptoms, we must test for more than TSH and T4. A full thyroid panel involves testing TSH, total T3, total T4, free T3, free T4, reverse T3, and thyroid antibodies.

Timing of testing is another important consideration. It is best to test in the morning when thyroid functioning is highest. This is because the thyroid functioning varies throughout the day (Kaczor 2012). If you retest your thyroid several months later, do that at the same time of the day to have a meaningful comparison of your results.

The last piece of evaluation needed is consideration of viruses and gut pathogens. This means testing for chronic viral load and other pathogens in the GI tract. We test how these might be negatively impacting your thyroid as well.

We cannot solely focus on the thyroid though. We must look at the whole body, including the adrenals, because if your thyroid is not doing the job, your adrenal glands pick up the slack.

ADRENAL

Your adrenals produce several important hormones, most notably stress hormones. You might be under a lot of stress in your daily life, so it is important to understand this dynamic. Modern lifestyle places excessive stress on your adrenals and can cause subclinical adrenal dysfunction.

What Do the Adrenals Do?

The adrenal glands are small, triangular-shaped glands located on top of your kidneys. They produce hormones that regulate:

- Metabolism
- Immune system
- Blood pressure
- Response to stress

Cortisol is a glucocorticoid hormone, which means it is a steroid hormone. In the short term and at low levels, it stimulates a healthy degree of inflammation. This ability to stimulate inflammation is beneficial because it helps our body heal itself. The problem arises when cortisol and the stress response persist over time. With persistent or higher levels of cortisol, inflammation is suppressed, as is the case with many steroids that are used in medicine. But when cortisol is persistently elevated over time, your body's ability to regulate inflammation and immune activity becomes dysfunctional (Yeager 2011, p. 333, Figure 1).

Stress is meant to be a short-lived and adaptive response. The problem arises when it persists over time. Cortisol increases blood sugar when you need to deal with a stressful situation. This is the sympathetic fight-or-flight response described earlier. Your body perceives a threat, so it prepares by moving sugar—energy—into your blood, so your muscles have fuel to run or fight.

For the same reason, cortisol also raises your blood pressure. It takes the body's focus away from bone formation, which can hurt our ability to form strong bones over time.

Finally, this hormone controls our sleep and wake cycles. Normally, cortisol rises and falls throughout the day in what is called a *diurnal cycle*—one that follows the cycle of increasing and decreasing light of day. It is higher in the morning to make you awake and alert enough to get out of bed. Later in the day, it begins to wane and finds its lowest level by bedtime.

Insulin is another hormone also responsible for regulating your blood sugar. Insulin is released from a different gland, the pancreas, helping your body regulate and utilize the sugar in your blood after you eat a meal. Insulin helps the energy to move from your blood into your cells, opening the door for the sugar to enter, so your cells have energy to use. If the stress response persists for too long, it can diminish insulin's ability to control your blood sugar.

We also have epinephrine and norepinephrine. These are what most people know as your adrenaline hormones. Like cortisol, these are part of the fight or flight stress response. These hormones activate during physically and emotionally stressful situations by increasing your heart rate and blood flow to your muscles and brain so you can respond to perceived threats. This is adaptive in the short term but can become harmful to your health in the long term.

Aldosterone is another hormone sending signals to your kidneys to regulate your blood pressure and electrolytes so your body can regulate the pH of the blood.

Lastly, DHEA is an androgenic steroid. DHEA is the precursor that converts to your sex hormones estrogen and testosterone. These are important, and we will talk more about them in the final section of this chapter.

Common Symptoms of Cortisol Dysfunction and Benefits of Correction

You have probably heard of *adrenal fatigue*, which is not actually a legitimate medical term. Though it is a commonly used colloquial phrase, *adrenal fatigue* is not the correct medical term for the referred symptom picture. This term is reserved for a more acutely severe form of disease. In fact, most people with stress or adrenal dysfunction do not actually have a medically recognized disease. Rather, the true cause of their symptoms will take some deeper digging.

The syndrome commonly referred to as *adrenal fatigue* is more accurately labeled *HPA axis dysregulation*. This happens when you have too much stress for too long and the *HPA axis*, the connection between your brain and adrenals, becomes unable to regulate healthy levels of cortisol.

As perceived stress persists for days and weeks, your adrenals produce too much cortisol, but as the perceived stress continues over months and years, the adrenals become exhausted and release less and less cortisol to the point of being deficient. Your body's ability to regulate the balance of cortisol becomes dysfunctional, leading to unregulated inflammation throughout the body.

This can lead to different issues depending on the individual:

- Arthritis
- Depression
- Chronic fatigue
- IBS
- Skin issues
- Crohn's disease
- Colitis

Inflammation is generally an underlying cause for all these conditions. The degree of inflammation present in the body largely depends on the hormone cortisol. Cortisol is anti-inflammatory, but only when levels are normal. It is when cortisol levels are too high or too low that the inflammatory balance is disturbed.

Increased stress and correspondingly high cortisol levels harm your body's ability to balance inflammation and regulate the immune response. Over time, your body is exposed to too much cortisol for too long, so your cells become less sensitive to the cortisol. In your body's attempt to fix this problem, your adrenals start working harder to pump out more cortisol. At this point, you might have excessive inflammation due to multiple stresses on your body, which is even more reason for your body to continue pumping out cortisol in an effort to control the damage and inflammation.

Symptoms resulting from excess cortisol production include:

- Fatigue
- Sleep problems
- Irritability
- Anxiety
- Feeling down or depressed
- Cravings for sugar, carbohydrates, fat, caffeine, and/ or salt
- Lack of afternoon energy
- Weight gain
- Getting sick more often
- Brain fog
- Forgetfulness
- Digestive problems

Other hormonal issues can occur since other endocrine glands are connected, such as the thyroid hormones. When you correct the dysfunction, you'll see the opposite of all things on the list above.

Over time the adrenals weaken, becoming tired from keeping up with cortisol demand, and alas, your cortisol levels dip too low. The levels will remain that way until the source of stress is removed and the body is given time to recover. At this point, you are feeling exhausted all the time, aches and pains are more stubborn, your ability to focus and get things done is impaired, and you may have put on quite a few pounds.

Prolonged stress, as discussed in the previous section, first increases levels of cortisol.

Hey, all you binge coffee drinkers! We are talking to you here. All that caffeine is going to stimulate your depleted adrenals to produce as much cortisol and adrenaline as they can. Because the adrenals are deficient at this point, this causes the tiredness that you feel after the initial energy boost from each cup.

As a result of the reduction in cortisol output, our body is also more likely to develop excessive inflammatory responses triggered by any other cause. There becomes less opposition to attack from bacteria, viruses, and toxins since your immune system has become weakened. The inflammation in your body surges as your immunity worsens.

Therefore, doctors often prescribe prednisone and hydrocortisone to suppress the immune response—steroid medications. This temporarily relieves symptoms, but its effects are short lived, and you must go back for repeated treatments. Many side effects can occur, and you can develop tissue damage, swelling, or weakened bones with long-term use.

You do not want to do that.

If you want to gain control over inflammation, especially if you have any of the concerns mentioned in this book, it is crucial for your body to have a balanced, constant supply of cortisol. Address the underlying stress response resulting in the excessive inflammation and dysfunctional immune system.

Insulin, as mentioned earlier, manages your blood sugar. When the stress causes your blood sugar to shoot up and down, especially if your adrenals are depleted and not pumping out enough adrenal hormones, you become chronically tired. As a result, many people try to adapt by eating more sugar and carbohydrates for an easy, quick energy fix. As a result, your body spikes its insulin level. Because sugar is absorbed so quickly by your body, the insulin level drops suddenly, and you feel tired again.

What do you do?

You reach for more easy energy in the form of sugar and carbs. Before you know it, your body is on an insulin roller coaster ride and the vicious cycle persists. So naturally that creates many of the same symptoms relative to the adrenal problems discussed.

Testing

Testing for insulin as a single marker is straightforward. These results can be combined with other common markers of blood sugar and inflammation dynamics like blood glucose,

Hemoglobin A1C, and hs-CRP, which is one of the markers for inflammation. Evaluation of adrenal function tends to be limited with most doctors. If they test, they test exclusively for cortisol using a single blood draw completed at one point during the day.

This is not enough. We need more comprehensive testing so we can paint the full picture. As we discussed, cortisol normally rises and falls in a diurnal rhythm, so testing must account for this. Instead of one single blood sample, multiple samples throughout the day are needed, typically collected at home through the saliva or urine.

Adrenal issues do not happen overnight, they develop over time, so it naturally requires patience to recover from it. As a rule, if you have mild fatigue due to adrenal imbalance, it may take three months to recover; moderate fatigue requires approximately six months, and severe fatigue, probably a year or more.

Finally, always make sure you see your conventional doctor so they can evaluate to rule out any other serious medical pathology that might be present.

REPRODUCTIVE

When people hear the word *hormones*, most think about reproductive hormones. These are primarily testosterone and estrogen. Testosterone is typically thought of as the male hormone, and estrogen the female hormone. In reality, males and females each carry both, albeit in different proportions. You need a balance of both hormones to give you good energy and libido, lift your moods, and feel that sense of overall vitality.

The changes in hormones that most women and men experience as they age have a lot to do with the dynamics of these sex hormones. Many women undergoing menopause experience significant changes and struggle to feel *like themselves again*. As a woman's reproductive ability nears its end, the ovaries' ability to produce these sex hormones decreases. The same goes for men; the testes' ability to produce these sex hormones decreases.

The gonads—the ovaries and testes—produce sex hormones in younger years. Fortunately, our adrenals continue to produce these sex hormones after the sex organs stop. This is another reason to take care of your adrenals: because they carry that production for the rest of your life.

What Do the Reproductive Hormones Do?

Each hormone gland relates to every other hormone gland. In the effort to restore balance to your body, we cannot regard sex hormones in isolation. We need to address the adrenals, the thyroid, your gut, and your liver, all together. The sex hormones are made by both the gonads and the adrenal glands. They are converted from other sex steroids in your fat tissue and other organs, like your liver.

Let us talk about estrogen. There are three forms of estrogen:

1. Estradiol.

   This is the strongest of the three forms. For a woman in her reproductive years, estradiol is the most abundant type of estrogen in the body. Its main function is for reproductive and fertility purposes. It promotes development of breast tissue, matures and releases the eggs, and thickens the uterus lining for implantation of fertilized eggs.

   It is also good for your skin, mood, brain, gut, mitochondria, immune system, and heart health. It also helps with your muscle function and bone density and helps you maintain a healthy weight. Many women gain weight during menopause due to a lack of estradiol, which can also cause poor bone health, osteoporosis, and mood swings. Too much can result in constipation, loss of sex drive, depression, and perhaps weight gain as well.

2. Estriol

   This hormone is mostly associated with pregnancy. The fetus and placenta create estriol when a woman is pregnant, in order to help sustain the pregnancy. Levels are highest three weeks before giving birth in order to prepare the body for this miraculous event.

3. Estrone

Estrone is the least powerful type of estrogen. It becomes predominate in later phases of life. Post-menopausal women have higher amounts of estrone. During your reproductive years, estradiol is the predominate hormone, but as you transition into menopause, estrone becomes the most common type of estrogen.

Progesterone is what women make after ovulation for fertility, but it also prevents osteoporosis, stroke, dementia, heart disease, and breast cancer. You need to have regular ovulatory cycles to have enough progesterone to benefit your health. Progesterone also acts a natural antidepressant. It enhances your mood, and it relieves anxiety. It has a calming effect on the brain by stimulating the brain's GABA receptors (Del Río et al. 2018).

GABA receptors are the neurotransmitters in your brain and nervous system that cause you to feel calm, peaceful, and worry-free. That is why anxiety surfaces when your progesterone levels are low. Progesterone also lowers inflammation. Progesterone keeps you calm, helps you sleep, and lowers inflammation. It converts to *allopregnanolone*, which is a steroid that also has a calming effect on the brain and decreases inflammation (Del Río et al. 2018; Balan et al. 2019; He et al. 2004).

Next is testosterone. In men, testosterone is responsible for libido, bone mass, fat distribution, and good muscle mass and strength. It is also for the production of red blood cells and for sperm. A small amount of testosterone is converted to estradiol, one of the forms of estrogen.

Do women need testosterone?

Yes, they do. Testosterone seems to conjure images of men with bulky muscles, aggression, and big libidos. Many believe women do not have to be concerned with testosterone, but this hormone is so much more than that.

It helps build strong bones, supports brain health, and increases energy and libido for women as well. It helps with weight loss, burning fat, and mood. So, a woman's body naturally produces testosterone, just as males' bodies do. Ultimately, for males and females, it is all about the balance between these hormones. Testosterone is as important for women's health as much as for men's.

Finally, we have *dehydroepiandrosterone*, more commonly known as DHEA, which is the most abundant adrenal steroid in the body. It is made by the adrenals, but then travels into cells throughout the body to be converted into testosterone and estrogen. This is the supply pool for your body to produce estrogen and testosterone as needed. The levels of DHEA depend on the individual's biochemistry, their age, and their gender. Natural levels of DHEA usually peak at age twenty-five and then decrease after that.

Common Symptoms and Benefits of Correction

For women, starting in your late thirties, your estrogen goes on a roller coaster ride. It fluctuates at some points, at times rising to almost three times higher than when you were younger. It can suddenly crash again. Month after month, it can rise and fall in a frustratingly unpredictable fashion. This especially happens as you get closer to menopause. This roller coaster ride can cause issues with menses, fertility, weight, mood, energy, skin, and more.

Now for the different types of hormonal imbalances. First is high estrogen, or what we call *estrogen excess*. High levels of estrogen can develop when the liver is not breaking down the estrogen properly. When the liver is not breaking estrogen down, it leads to a backup in estrogen processing in the body, which results in higher-than-normal levels. There is not enough progesterone to counterbalance the elevated estrogen, so estrogen becomes predominate. This, in turn, creates a proportionately lower amount of progesterone.

This causes estrogen excess conditions, such as:

- Endometriosis
- Breast cancer
- Ovarian cancer
- Systemic inflammation

There is a direct link between inflammation and *aromatase activity*. Aromatase is present in fat tissue and is an enzyme responsible for regulating the amount of estrogen. And when there is increased aromatase activity, there is also increased chronic inflammation (Morris et al. 2011; Monteiro, Teixeira, and Calhau1 2014).

This is a vicious cycle because the chronic inflammation activates the aromatase, then the aromatase subsequently increases the production of estrogen in fat tissue. Increased estrogen then causes the body to store more fat. Fat tissue is also inflammatory and produces even more estrogen. The resulting inflammation then triggers aromatase, and around and around the cycle we go.

This increased estrogen can cause problems with your blood sugar—a condition we call *insulin resistance.* Estrogen deficiency can cause this as well. It also interrupts the satiation messages of your leptin, promoting obesity. Obesity means increased fat tissue, more inflammation, more estrogen production via aromatase, adding to the vicious cycle (Picon-Ruiz et al. 2017).

Other concerns that can result from this dynamic are:

- Endometriosis
- PMS
- Breast pain
- Painful, heavy periods
- Irritable mood
- Fluid retention
- Weight gain

Symptoms of high estrogen that are not addressed create more risk for hormonal cancers, especially:

- Breast cancer (Travis and Key 2003; Morris et al. 2011; Brown 2017)
- Autoimmune disease (Cutolo et al. 2006)
- Candida overgrowth (Wira et al. 2010)
- Hashimoto's disease and other thyroid issues (Santin and Furlanetto 2011)

In men, excess estrogen can cause breast development, sexual dysfunction, and infertility.

Symptoms of low estrogen can include:

- Night sweats
- Depression
- Weight gain
- Hot flashes
- Vaginal dryness
- Insomnia
- Incontinence
- Hair loss

You can substantially replenish your estrogen levels in the form of hormone replacement; however, depending on your circumstances, it is not always the safest route to go. After menopause, it can be difficult to help your ovaries start making more estrogen again, but there are supportive nutrients and herbs that can assist. It is also important to make sure the estrogen you do have is being processed and utilized in the body properly. Addressing all of your other hormonal glands will aid this process as well.

If you experience low estrogen but are not in menopause, the cause must be discovered. That means addressing disruptions to your estrogen, such as environmental toxins, psychosomatic stress, and detox issues and evaluating other medical conditions.

Low progesterone relates to stress because your body always chooses survival through stress over the calming and reproductive effects of progesterone. When you are exposed to chronic stress, the cortisol produced will be detrimental to progesterone activity.

Low progesterone can also be related to other hormonal issues like hypothyroidism, PCOS, or estrogen excess, so we need to evaluate for those as well. After age thirty-five there is an inevitable decline in progesterone. As you approach menopause, you ovulate less frequently, and your body produces less progesterone when you do ovulate. Some symptoms of low progesterone include:

- Cystic breasts
- Mid-cycle spotting
- Anxiety
- Insomnia
- Irritability

- Menstrual cramps
- Heavy menses

Low testosterone is associated with an increase in metabolic disease, meaning obesity, insulin resistance, and abnormal lipids or cholesterol levels, all of which often culminate in type 2 diabetes (Muraleedharan and Jones 2010). Presence of low testosterone and such metabolic syndromes are not only associated with increased risk of death from a cardiovascular event, but also overall risk of death due to *any* cause. With low testosterone also develops systemic inflammation (Friedrich 2011).

Testosterone plays a role in this by decreasing production of inflammatory molecules in your body. Lack of testosterone also increases inflammation via lack of muscle growth. Since we already know that muscle creates anti-inflammatory mediators while fat tissue does the opposite, having a low ratio of muscle to fat tissue in your body because of low testosterone will allow inflammation to develop unopposed.

Because testosterone already decreases naturally as we age, you need to optimize your ability to burn fat and build muscle to make sure you don't put, or keep on, that unwanted weight. All of this explains why symptoms of low testosterone are fatigue, depression, disinterest in sex, memory loss, and joint pain.

Testing

If you think you have a hormone imbalance, then testing is crucial. Knowing the nature and extent of the imbalance will determine how to properly treat it.

Testosterone and SHBG

A comprehensive exploration of testosterone involves both total testosterone and free testosterone, as well as *sex hormone binding globulin* (SHBG), a blood transfer protein for testosterone and estrogen.

Ninety-eight percent of the testosterone in your body is bound to proteins, either SHBG or albumin. This is what we call *bound testosterone*. The other 2 percent in your body is called *free testosterone* because it is not bound to proteins. Because it is unbound, free testosterone can connect with the cell receptors throughout your body. When a cell absorbs the testosterone, which might be a bone or muscle cell, it utilizes free testosterone to enable that cell's function.

Total testosterone is what the name suggests, the total of all testosterone hormones in your bloodstream. While your total testosterone levels might appear healthy, you could still have dysfunctional levels of free and active testosterone and SHBG. That is why we need a deeper look. Testosterone can be tested any time of the day or month but is best done in the morning when it is the highest. The sample can be taken via blood, urine, or saliva.

DHEA

DHEA, the crucial anti-aging hormone that converts to estrogen or testosterone, can be tested at any time of the month. This is typically done along with cortisol testing.

Estrogen and Progesterone

If you are still menstruating, then you want to check out estradiol. If you are post-menopausal, we may want to check estrone in addition to estradiol. Remember, estrone is the more predominate form of estrogen present after menopause. Estrogen must be tested based on the timing of your cycle.

Conventionally, you're directed to get your blood drawn for estrogen tests any day you are able to. Instead, to get an accurate and full picture, samples must be gathered at a specific time of your cycle. Day three of your cycle is the best time to test estradiol as well as FSH (follicle stimulating hormone) and LH (luteinizing hormone), which are hormones that work alongside estrogen.

Progesterone

Your body makes more progesterone during the second half of your cycle following ovulation, also called the *luteal phase*. You want to test progesterone levels when they should be the highest, generally about 5–7 days after ovulation. Essentially, that means testing sometime between days 19–22 of your cycle, assuming you have a 28-day cycle. If you are postmenopausal, the timing isn't as important; progesterone can be tested anytime.

While men also have progesterone, testing is not typically relevant.

Action Item

- *We recommend getting a full hormone evaluation that will ultimately be necessary to pinpoint your unique imbalance, if there is any, so that appropriate recommendations can be provided.*

- *For now, focus on applying all the previously mentioned action items, as every other Pillar has a substantial influence on your hormonal balance.*

Conclusion

Congratulations!

Because you have finished this book, here is what you should know:

- People in this country are not getting any better and instead are becoming sicker.

- The current healthcare system fails to address the real cause of common issues.

- There is a different approach to wellness—a functional approach—that uses the necessary foundations of health that determine the difference between a healthy, vibrant life and an unwell, suppressed one.

If you have been struggling, whether for a few months or a lifetime, know you are not alone. Your situation is not your fault. It is fundamentally a product of a failed healthcare system. To find success, you need a better approach. Albert Einstein is often credited with having said it best: *Insanity is doing the same thing over and over and expecting different results.*

Most importantly, you understand your health is either getting better or worse, never staying the same. And because you are not a victim of your health, but a creator of it, you know you can use the Pillars of Health as your tool to put yourself on the right path going forward. The factors that determine your level of health—or disease—are in your control.

Recall Caron in the first chapter.

She was the woman who turned around her sleep, energy, and digestive issues, and now looks forward to each day rather than dreading it. Not only did she escape the limitations of ill health and turn her life around, but she also saw the immense value in empowering herself to become independent with her health. This way she no longer had to be dependent on over-the-counter drugs to manage her symptoms and to push herself through each and every day.

She says, "Now that I know how to feel better, I am committed to continuing this healthy lifestyle; knowing even if I slip occasionally, I have the knowledge and the tools to self-correct."

This is how you can learn to become your own doctor, rather than relying on doctors or medications for the rest of your life. That is not to say a health issue will never come up again, but it is to say you will know how to handle it if something *does* come up. Once you understand the concepts delivered in this book, you and your healthcare team must apply them to your unique situation.

To summarize, let's cover the five steps of what it means to take that path:

1. Discern the right purpose.

   It is essential to be honest with yourself about your current situation. Acknowledge what concerns you have about your current path. Once you've developed clarity about this, develop your *why* by envisioning what you want life to be like instead. Only then can you sincerely commit to move toward the life that you desire.

2. Determine the true cause of your current concerns.

   Determining the true cause necessitates using the correct testing and evaluation. The best way to do this is working with a trained professional—someone who takes time to learn about your unique situation to help you figure out the true underlying cause of your individual concerns.

3. Treat the cause.

   Once the cause has been determined, you can correct it. Medication does not treat the cause. If you have high cholesterol, the medication does not actually resolve the problem and may present side effects as well. Instead, a comprehensive lifestyle approach will address the true underlying cause and minimize potential side effects.

4. Use a proven system to address the cause within a larger holistic approach.

I have discussed how most failure results from not having a system. Most of the practice members we work with have all tried many things before, and we are usually not the first stop on their healthcare journey. They have put the effort in and may have even tried to implement one or two of the Pillars from this book, so their failure is not the result of lack of effort.

Rather it is because they did not implement all the Pillars together at the same time, in a stepwise and individualized approach. They have simply followed the wrong path. Nearly every time, the problem was that they were not treating the whole body in an individualized way or using a comprehensive system.

You can get a head start on this by doing the action items mentioned at the end of each chapter. Start with one change until it feels easy, and then add succeeding changes. This will start the process of putting your overall wellness and vitality on track.

5. Find a mentor.

It is crucial to find an expert to guide you to where you want to be, someone who has walked that path before and can show you the way. Musicians, athletes, or other experts in their fields have mentors or coaches helping them climb the ladder of success. They started at a place below their ultimate goal and had coaches to teach and empower them with what they needed to find success.

At Nature Medicine Clinic, we are not traditional doctors—we are not here to *fix* you. Instead, we serve as your mentors to guide you down the path toward greater health. Ultimately you are the one who must walk the path. We cannot do that for you, but we will support you the entire way.

Whenever we sit down for a wellness consultation with someone, there are a few key steps. After we acquire a comprehensive health history and look at lab results, we always ask a series of questions:

1. If you could paint the picture of perfect health, what would that look like?

2. If you stay on your current path and do not make any changes, what are your fears and concerns about where that path might lead you?

3. If we can help you to get to that perfect picture of health, are you prepared to make the appropriate lifestyle changes necessary to achieve your health goals?

I invite you, the reader, to consider these questions for yourself. Now that you have read through the entirety of this book, answer these questions:

- If you stay on your current path, where exactly will it lead?

- If the path concerns you, then where do you want to be instead?

- Are you willing and ready to do what is required to get to your destination?

- Do you have the right support to help you get there?

In this line of work, we witness many people making incredible transformations in their lives and health. Regrettably, we also see many who decide to procrastinate. Procrastination is the greatest sorrow because it completely evades any opportunity for you to change. You are not like a cat with nine lives; you only have this one life to live.

People procrastinate for many reasons. Maybe you are afraid to make changes. Maybe you don't believe that you need to do anything different and that your health will just sort itself out one day. Or maybe you think you'll just do it later or you feel good enough just knowing that you read this book.

Ultimately, these people all end up in the same place, not taking any action. Sometimes we see them six months down the road, and all too often, their health is worse. It pains me to see those people because I know if they had made a different decision earlier, they would have ended up in a much better place today.

So just know that we are here to support you unconditionally. There is always room for you to make improvements with your health, whether you are just looking to optimize your health, are taking ten or more medications with severe health concerns, or fall anywhere in between.

While many people are stuck thinking about their health and not doing anything about it, my hope is that you will be the exception—that you will be part of the minority who acts and creates change toward the life you desire.

If what you have read resonates with you, then my hope is that you take the first step. I invite you to imagine yourself achieving greater health and a greater life. If that vision ignites a fire in you and you want to commit, then there are two things you must do:

1. You must participate in the process.

2. You must find and work with a mentor.

To help you accomplish this, I offer you this opportunity to participate in your transformation and receive mentorship.

Action item

- *For us to get to know you better, we invite you to sit down with one of our doctors for a comprehensive, one-on-one consultation to discuss your health concerns, and your health goals, all so that we can customize a plan of action for you.*

- *We have a special offer for anyone who has read this book. To learn more about that, call our office and we will be happy to help you take the very first step to taking control of your health.*

While a journey of a thousand miles begins with a single step, the first step is the most difficult. Many have a hard time committing to themselves and their health journey. When that does happen, it is almost always that very first step, getting started.

This first step may involve some growing pains, but it comes with the recognition that this health journey of a thousand steps will last the rest of your life. It will provide you the long-term freedom of everlasting health. Your health journey is about evolving into the best version of yourself, and it is for you to decide if you are worth that.

We are here for you to lean on for those first few difficult steps and through the rest of the process, even for the rest of your life.

Next Steps

If you'd like to pursue this opportunity for greater health, give our office a call at 561-571-3326 or scan the QR code below. We have a special offer for you after reading this book.

References

American Medical Association. "Trends in Health Care Spending." ama-assn.org/about/research/trends-health-care-spending.

Amino, Nobuyuki. 1988. "4 Autoimmunity and Hypothyroidism." *Baillière's Clinical Endocrinology and Metabolism* 2, no. 3: 591–617. doi.org/10.1016/S0950-351X(88)80055-7.

Andrew, D. 2018. "94 Percent Chance It's a System Failure, Not You." *Medium.com.* April 16, 2018. medium.com/the-mission/whos-to-blame-94-chance-it-s-a-system-failure-not-you-26396b2b38110055-7.

Balan, Irina, Matthew C. Beattie, Todd K. O'Buckley, Laure Aurelian, and A. Leslie Morrow. 2019. "Endogenous Neurosteroid (3α,5α)3-Hydroxypregnan-20-one Inhibits Toll-like-4 Receptor Activation and Pro-inflammatory Signaling in Macrophages and Brain." *Scientific Reports* 9, article 1220. doi.org/10.1038/s41598-018-37409-6.

Ballarini, Tommaso, Debora Melo van Lent, Julia Brunner, Alina Schröder, Steffen Wolfsgruber, Slawek Altenstein, Frederic Brosseron, Katharina Buerger, Peter Dechent, Laura Dobisch, Emrah Düzel, Birgit Ertl-Wagner, Klaus Fliessbach, Silka Dawn

Freiesleben, Ingo Frommann, Wenzel Glanz, Dietmar Hauser, John Dylan Haynes, Michael T. Heneka, Daniel Janowitz, Ingo Kilimann, Christoph Laske, Franziska Maier, Coraline Danielle Metzger, Matthias H. Munk, Robert Perneczky, Oliver Peters, Josef Priller, Alfredo Ramirez, Boris-Stephan Rauchmann, Nina Roy, Klaus Scheffler, Anja Schneider, Annika Spottke, Eike Jakob Spruth, Stefan J. Teipel, Ruth Vukovich, Jens Wiltfang, Frank Jessen, and Michael Wagner. 2021. "Mediterranean Diet, Alzheimer Disease Biomarkers, and Brain Atrophy in Old Age." *Neurology* 96, no. 24. n.neurology.org/content/96/24/e2920.

Blom, Wendy A., Anne Lluch, Annette Stafleu, Sophie Vinoy, Jens J. Holst, Gertjan Schaafsma, and Henk F. J. Hendriks. 2006. "Effect of a High-Protein Breakfast on the Postprandial Ghrelin Response." *Am J Clin Nutr* 83, no. 2: 211–20. doi.org/10.1093/ajcn/83.2.211.

Brown, Kristy A, Neil M. Iyengar, Xi Kathy Zhou, Ayca Gucalp, Kotha Subbaramaiah, Hanhan Wang, Dilip D. Giri, Monica Morrow, Domenick J. Falcone, Nils K. Wendel, Lisle A. Winston, Michael Pollak, Anneloor Dierickx, Clifford A. Hudis, and Andrew J. Dannenberg. 2017. "Menopause Is a Determinant of Breast Aromatase Expression and Its Associations With BMI, Inflammation, and Systemic Markers." *The*

Journal of Clinical Endocrinology & Metabolism 102, no. 5: 1692–1701. doi.org/10.1210/jc.2016-3606.

Buttorff Christine, T. Ruder, and M. Bauman. 2017. *Multiple Chronic Conditions in the United States.* Santa Monica, CA: Rand Corp.

Centers for Disease Control and Prevention A. "Chronic Diseases in America." cdc.gov/chronicdisease/resources/infographic/chronic-diseases.htm.

Centers for Disease Control and Prevention B. "Poor Nutrition." cdc.gov/chronicdisease/pdf/factsheets/poor-nutrition-H.pdf.

Cole, Greg M., Qiu-Lan Ma, and Sally A. Frautschy. 2009. "Omega-3 Fatty Acids and Dementia." *Prostaglandins, Leukotrienes & Essential Fatty Acids* 81, no. 2–3: 213–221. doi.org/10.1016/j.plefa.2009.05.015.

Cutolo, Maurizio, Silvia Capellino, Alberto Sulli, Bruno Serioli, Maria Elena Secchi, Barbara Villaggio, and Rainer H. Straub. 2006. "Estrogens and Autoimmune Diseases." *Annals of the New York Academy of Sciences*, no. 1089: 538–547. 10.1196/annals.1386.043.

Del Río, Juan Pablo, María I. Alliende, Natalia Molina, Felipe G. Serrano, Santiago Molina, and Pilar Vigil. 2018. "Steroid Hormones and Their Action in Women's Brains: The Importance of Hormonal

Balance." *Frontiers in Public Health* 6:141. doi. org/10.3389/fpubh.2018.00141.

Friedrich Schiller University–Jena. 2011. "How Testosterone Protects Against Inflammation." *Science Daily*. sciencedaily.com/ releases/2011/07/110726093146.htm.

Furman, David. 2019. "Chronic Inflammation in the Etiology of Disease Across the Life Span." *Nature Medicine* 25: 1822–1832. doi.org/10.1038/s41591-019-0675-0.

Garber, Jeffery R., Rhoda H. Cobin, Hossein Gharib, James V. Hennessey, Irwin Klein, Jeffrey I. Mechanick, Rachel Pessah-Pollack, Peter A. Singer, and Kenneth A. Woeber. 2012. "Clinical Practice Guidelines for Hypothyroidism in Adults: Cosponsored by the American Association of Clinical Endocrinologists and the American Thyroid Association." *Endocrine Practice* 18, no. 6: 817–1041. doi.org/10.4158/EP12280.GL.

He, Jun, Chheng-Orn Evans, Stuart W. Hoffman, Nelson M. Oyesiku, and Donald G. Stein. 2004. "Progesterone and Allopregnanolone Reduce Inflammatory Cytokines After Traumatic Brain Injury." *Experimental Neurology* 189, no. 2: 404–412. doi.org/10.1016/j. expneurol.2004.06.008.

Hunter, Philip. 2012. "The Inflammation Theory of Disease." *EMBO reports* 13, no. 11. doi.org/10.1038/embor.2012.142.

Jara, Evelyn L., Natalia Muñoz-Durango, Carolina Llanos, Natalia Muñoz-Durango, Carolina Llanos, Carlos Fardella, Pablo A. González, Susan M. Bueno, Alexis M. Kalergis, and Claudia A. Riedel. 2017. "Modulating the Function of the Immune System by Thyroid Hormones and Thyrotropin." *Immunology Letters* 184: 76–83. doi.org/10.1016/j.imlet.2017.02.010.

Javaheri, Sogol, Shahrokh Javaheri, and Ali Javaheri. 2013. "Sleep Apnea, Heart Failure, and Pulmonary Hypertension." *Curr Heart Fail Rep* 10: 315–320. doi.org/10.1007/s11897-013-0167-3.

Kaczor, Tina. 2012. "Thyroid-Stimulating Hormone Fluctuates With Time of Day." *Natural Medicine Journal* 4, no. 12. naturalmedicinejournal.com/journal/2012-12/thyroid-stimulating-hormone-fluctuates-time-day.

Kasasbeh, E., David S. Chi, and G. Krishnaswamy. 2006. "Inflammatory Aspects of Sleep Apnea and Their Cardiovascular Consequences." *Southern Medical Association* 99, no. 1: 58–67. doi.org/10.1097/01.smj.0000197705.99639.50.

Knutson, Kristen L., Armand M. Ryden, Bryce A. Mander, and Eve Van Cauter. 2006. "Role of Sleep Duration and Quality in the Risk and Severity of Type 2 Diabetes Mellitus." *Arch Intern Med*, no.166: 1768–1764. doi.org/10.1001/archinte.166.16.1768.

Ma, Yanjun, Lirong Liang, Fanfan Zheng, Le Shi, Bao-Liang Zhong, and Wuxiang Xie. 2020. "Association Between Sleep Duration and Cognitive Decline." *JAMA Network Open*. doi.org/10.1001/jamanetworkopen.2020.13573.

Martin, Ann B., M. Hartman, D. Lassman, and A. Catlin. 2020. "National Health Care Spending In 2019: Steady Growth For The Fourth Consecutive Year." *Health Aff.* 40, no.1 :1–11. doi.org/10.1377/hlthaff.2020.02022.

Monteiro, Rosário, Diana Teixeira, and Conceição Calhau1. 2014. "Estrogen Signaling in Metabolic Inflammation." *Mediators of Inflammation*. doi.org/10.1155/2014/615917.

Morris, Patrick G., Clifford A. Hudis, Dilip Giri, Monica Morrow, Domenick J. Falcone, Xi Kathy Zhou, Baoheng Du, Edi Brogi, Carolyn B. Crawford, Levy Kopelovich, Kotha Subbaramaiah, and Andrew J. Dannenberg. 2011. "Inflammation and Increased Aromatase Expression Occur in the Breast Tissue of Obese Women with Breast Cancer." *Cancer Prev Res*

4: 1021–1029. doi.org/10.1158/1940-6207.CAPR-11-0110.

Mullington, Janet M., Norah S. Simpson, Hans K. Meier-Ewert, and Monika Haack. 2010. "Sleep Loss and Inflammation." *Best Practice & Research Clinical Endocrinology & Metabolism* 24, no. 5: 775–784. doi.org/10.1016/j.beem.2010.08.014.

Muñoz-Garach, Araceli, Beatriz García-Fontana, and Manuel Muñoz-Torres. 2020. "Nutrients and Dietary Patterns Related to Osteoporosis." *Nutrients* 12, no. 7. doi.org/10.3390/nu12071986.

Muraleedharan, Vakkat and T. Hugh Jones. 2010. "Review: Testosterone and the metabolic syndrome." *Therapeutic Advances in Endocrinology and Metabolism*, no. 1: 207–223. doi.org/10.1177/2042018810390258.

Nunn, Ryan. 2020. "A Dozen Facts About the Economics of the U.S. Health-Care System." brookings.edu/research/a-dozen-facts-about-the-economics-of-the-u-s-health-care-system.

Picon-Ruiz, Manuel, Cynthia Morata-Tarifa, Janeiro J. Valle-Goffin, Eitan R. Friedman, and Joyce M. Slingerland. 2017. "Obesity and Adverse Breast Cancer Risk and Outcome: Mechanistic Insights and Strategies for Intervention." *CA: A Cancer Journal for Clinicians* 67, no. 5: 378–397. doi.org/10.3322/caac.21405.

Ruesten, Anne Von, Cornelia Weikert, Ingo Fietze, and Heiner Boeing. 2012. "Association of Sleep Duration with Chronic Diseases in the European Prospective Investigation into Cancer and Nutrition (EPIC)-Potsdam Study." *PLOS ONE.* doi.org/10.1371/journal.pone.0030972.

Santin, Ana Paula, and Tania Weber Furlanetto. 2011. "Role of Estrogen in Thyroid Function and Growth Regulation." *Journal of Thyroid Research*, no. 2011. doi.org/10.4061/2011/875125.

Schneider, Eric C. et al. 2021. *"Mirror, Mirror 2021—Reflecting Poorly: Health Care in the U.S. Compared to Other High-Income Countries."* (Commonwealth Fund Aug. 2021). doi.org/10.26099/01dv-h208.

Schug, Thaddeus T., Amanda Janesick, Bruce Blumberg, and Jerrold J. Heindela. 2011. "Endocrine Disrupting Chemicals and Disease Susceptibility." *The Journal of Steroid Biochemistry and Molecular Biology* 127, no. 3–5: 204–215. doi.org/10.1016/j.jsbmb.2011.08.007.

Shahid, Muhammad A., Muhammad A. Ashraf, and Sandeep Sharma. 2022. "Physiology, Thyroid Hormone." *StatPearls Publishing.* ncbi.nlm.nih.gov/books/NBK500006/.

Shokri-Kojori, Ehsan, Gene-Jack Wang, Corinde E. Wiers, and Nora D. Volkow. 2018. "β-Amyloid

Accumulation in the Human Brain After One Night of Sleep Deprivation." *Proceedings of the National Academy of Sciences*, 115. doi.org/10.1073/pnas.1721694115.

Taheri, S. 2006. "The Link Between Short Sleep Duration and Obesity: We should Recommend More Sleep to Prevent Obesity." *Arch Dis Child*, 91:881–884. dx.doi.org/10.1136/adc.2005.093013.

Taheri, Shahrad, Ling Lin, Diane Austin, Terry Young, and Emmanuel Mignot. 2004. "Short Sleep Duration is Associated with Reduced Leptin, Elevated Ghrelin, and Increased Body Mass Index." *PLOS Medicine*. doi.org/10.1371/journal.pmed.0010062.

Thomas, J., C. J. Thomas, J. Radcliffe, and C. Itsiopoulos. 2015. "Omega-3 Fatty Acids in Early Prevention of Inflammatory Neurodegenerative Disease: A Focus on Alzheimer's Disease." *BioMed Research International*, vol. 2015, Article ID 172801. doi.org/10.1155/2015/172801.

Tinker A. 2017. "How to Improve Patient Outcomes for Chronic Diseases and Comorbidities." healthcatalyst.com/wp-content/uploads/2014/04/How-to-Improve-Patient-Outcomes.pdf.

Travis, Ruth C. and Timothy J. Key. 2003. "Oestrogen Exposure and Breast Cancer Risk." *Breast Cancer Research* 5, no 239. doi.org/10.1186/bcr628.

Weigle, David S, Patricia A Breen, Colleen C. Matthys, Holly S. Callahan, Kaatje E. Meeuws, Verna R. Burden, and Jonathan Q. Purnell. 2005. "A High-Protein Diet Induces Sustained Reductions in Appetite, ad Libitum Caloric Intake, and Body Weight Despite Compensatory Changes in Diurnal Plasma Leptin and Ghrelin Concentrations." *The American Journal of Clinical Nutrition*, 82, no. 1: 41–48. doi.org/10.1093/ajcn/82.1.41.

Wira, Charles R, John V. Fahey, Mimi Ghosh, Mickey V. Patel, Danica K. Hickey, and Daniel O. Ochiel. 2010. "Review Article: Sex Hormone Regulation of Innate Immunity in the Female Reproductive Tract: The Role of Epithelial Cells in Balancing Reproductive Potential with Protection Against Sexually Transmitted Pathogens." *American Journal of Reproductive Immunology*, no. 63: 544–565. doi.org/10.1111/j.1600-0897.2010.00842.x.

Yeager, Mark P. et al. 2011. "Cortisol Exerts Bi-phasic Regulation of Inflammation in Humans." *Dose-Response : A Publication of International Hormesis Society* vol. 9.3: 332-47. doi:10.2203/dose-response.10-013.Yeager

Zimmerman M., J. B. McGlinchey, D. Young, and I. Chelminski. 2006. "Diagnosing Major Depressive Disorder I: A Psychometric Evaluation of the DSM-IV

Symptom Criteria." *J Nerv Ment Dis* 2006, 194:158–163. pubmed.ncbi.nlm.nih.gov/16534432/.

About the Authors

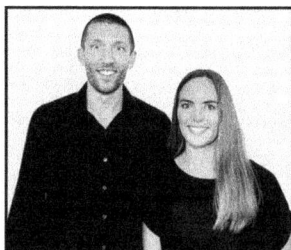

Husband and wife, Adam and Krista are Naturopathic Doctors. They help people take control of their health to reverse chronic disease. Having worked with thousands of patients to do exactly this, they continue to be inspired by witnessing many lives completely transform, and this fuels their mission.

Naturopathic medicine became the natural choice for Dr. Krista after she struggled with *Polycystic Ovarian Syndrome* at a young age and was told all she could do was take medications for life. Having been raised in a family full of conventional doctors, she realized that something important was missing from the current medical system—hope.

Dr. Adam spent several months in China on a medical internship and was blown away by the contrasting healthcare crisis in the United States. This crisis was also evidenced by the lack of improvement in his father's condition after he was debilitated by chronic disease following the 9/11 disaster in New York City. Recognizing that there was more to health than pills and procedures, Dr. Adam pursued medicine that could empower people rather than leave them stuck on the hamster wheel of conventional medicine.

These two doctors met during their training at the National University of Natural Medicine. Their additional training in acupuncture and Ayurvedic medicine complements their holistic perspective on wellness. Together they have contributed to the holistic medicine research base by publishing two case reports in an integrative medicine journal. They are simultaneously fluent in conventional medicine and biomedical training, which empowers their practice members to take control of their healing. This mélange of natural therapies is transferred to their practice members, so members feel less *stuck* and more *free* to live the life they desperately want to live.

www.ingramcontent.com/pod-product-compliance
Lightning Source LLC
Chambersburg PA
CBHW071851200326
41519CB00016B/4329